1

Financial management and resource management

AIMS

This chapter highlights the need for good financial management in the modern NHS and aims to:

- explain the link between the provision of funding and the resources this is used to acquire;
- identify the resources used in the provision of health care: staff; assets, facilities and consumables; information and information systems; and finance;
- outline the constraints within which resources have to be managed;
- describe the various ways, over the years, in which value for money has been sought in the NHS;
- trace the development of financial management in the NHS so as to put current practices in their historical context.

The need for good financial management

Everyone employed in the NHS is to some extent involved in financial management, some through formal arrangements, and others, perhaps without realizing it, through their routine contribution to the health care process. This involvement has seen a marked increase in recent years and there is little doubt that it will continue to grow and spread to include a wider spectrum of staff at increasingly lower levels.

Those attempting to gain an appropriate understanding of financial management frequently fail to realize that it is not just a matter of checking every so often that the total pounds and pence spent last week/month/year was as expected. Simply knowing how much was spent does not automatically lead to good financial management. Rather, this requires knowing much more about the finances being managed, such as: 'why, where, how, by whom, when, on what . . . was the money spent?' Answering these questions requires an understanding of resource provision and consumption, and a comprehension as to why resources have to be managed and how this can be accomplished. Resource management is inextricably linked with financial management; the theoretical and practical aspects of this link provide a common theme throughout this book.

Funding and resource management

The money, or funding, allocated to the NHS is provided for the purpose of acquiring the resources deemed necessary and suitable for the provision of health care, either directly or indirectly. Money in itself is of no benefit; the benefit is derived from what can be acquired and achieved with its use.

Each year, the NHS is given a fixed amount of money to spend on the provision of health care, with the effect that the volume and type of resources that can be acquired and used are limited. Resource consumption has therefore to be planned carefully, and actual resource consumption then controlled against these plans to ensure that the available funding is not exceeded. Planning and control should exist in any situation where the achievement of goals, objectives or outcomes is required, and the design and maintenance of the planning and control processes, the provision of the required information and its correct use are all essential if control is to be applied successfully. The level of this success is normally dependent on the result of one or more decisions, the validity of which in turn are dependent upon adequate and appropriate information being available in the correct place and at the correct time.

The methods and processes used to ensure that the rate and level of financial spend are controlled are described by the generic term **financial management**. Since funding is used simply to obtain resources, it therefore follows that it is the rate and level of resource consumption that must be controlled if finance is to be controlled. This requires resource management as well as financial management.

Thus, managing finance is all about managing resources and one important responsibility of management is to ensure the efficient and effective use of resources, regardless of funding levels. It may be argued that the need for tight financial management and control arises solely because finance is limited, and that, if a greater level of funding were provided to the NHS, the need for such control would diminish or even disappear. However, this is not so. No matter how great or how small the total level of funding available, it is essential that resources are consumed in such a way that the purpose for which that level of funding was provided is achieved to the fullest possible extent, i.e. with maximum efficiency and effectiveness. Even if funding were open-ended, the responsibility to ensure its effective and efficient use would still exist because there are many competing demands for public funds.

Many consider that there is a basic underfunding issue within the NHS that needs to be addressed, and that current financial and resource management techniques do nothing to resolve this. Claims that the NHS is underfunded, with an associated implication that this is the sole cause of the need to control spending, have been

PAMs	Professions Allied to Medicine
PAS	patient administration system
PDC	public dividend capital
PES	public expenditure survey
PMS	patient management system
PI	performance indicator
PSBR	Public Sector Borrowing Requirement
Pt.	patient
QALY	quality-adjusted life year
RAWG	Resource Allocation Working Group
RAWP	Resource Allocation Working Party
RCCS	revenue consequences of capital schemes
RGN	registered general nurse
RHA	regional health authority
RM	resource management
RMI	Resource Management Initiative
SCRAW	Steering Committee for Resource Allocation in Wales
SFIs	standing financial instructions
SHA	special health authority
SHARE	Scottish Health Authorities Revenue Equalization
SHO	senior house officer
SIFTR	Service Increment for Teaching and Research
SIS	supplies information system
SPS	standard payroll system
SSAP	Statement of Standard Accounting Practice
UGM	unit general manager
VAT	value added tax
VFM	value for money
WTE	whole time equivalent
ZBB	zero-based budgeting
£k	thousands of pounds
£m	millions of pounds

Financial Management in the NHS

Financial Management in the NHS
A manager's handbook

Howard Mellett

Cardiff Business School
Cardiff

Neil Marriott

Cardiff Business School
Cardiff

and

Stephen Harries

Executive Director of Finance
Llandough Hospital NHS Trust
Cardiff

CHAPMAN & HALL

University and Professional Division

London · Glasgow · New York · Tokyo · Melbourne · Madras

Published by Chapman & Hall, 2–6 Boundary Row, London SE1 8HN, UK

Chapman & Hall, 2–6 Boundary Row, London SE1 8HN, UK

Blackie Academic & Professional, Wester Cleddens Road, Bishopbriggs, Glasgow G64 2NZ, UK

Chapman & Hall Inc., One Penn Plaza, 41st Floor, New York NY10119, USA

Chapman & Hall Japan, Thomson Publishing Japan, Hirakawacho Nemoto Building, 6F, 1-7-11 Hirakawa-cho, Chiyoda-ku, Tokyo 102, Japan

Chapman & Hall Australia, Thomas Nelson Australia, 102 Dodds Street, South Melbourne, Victoria 3205, Australia

Chapman & Hall India, R. Seshadri, 32 Second Main Road, CIT East, Madras 600 035, India

First edition 1993

© 1993 Howard Mellett, Neil Marriott and Stephen Harries

Typeset in $9\frac{1}{2}/11\frac{1}{2}$ pt Meridien by Excel Typesetters Company, Hong Kong
Printed in England by Clays Ltd, St Ives PLC

ISBN 0 412 47320 8

A catalogue record for this book is available from the British Library

Library of Congress Cataloging-in-Publication data available

∞ Printed on permanent acid-free text paper, manufactured in accordance with the proposed ANSI/NISO Z 39.48-199X and ANSI Z 39.48-1984

To Catherine, Elizabeth, Hannah and Alexander

Contents

Preface

This book has been written as a partnership between a practitioner with substantial NHS experience and two academics who have had a long-term interest in NHS financial management. This blend has resulted in a book that brings out the best of both worlds, as it provides the necessary theoretical underpinning to enable the procedures described to be applied in a variety of local situations, and also sets this theory in a context which NHS staff are familiar with.

The reforms in the NHS which took place in the early 1990s resulted in a fundamental overhaul of its financial management. Managerial decisions and their financial consequences have come under closer scrutiny than ever before, and more and more of those involved in the health care process have had to become financially aware. At the same time, the creation of health care providers as separate entities, the NHS trusts, means that the success or failure of an individual facility depends on its own performance. Many managers have been trained as specialists in areas other than finance, but they now rely on financial information and its interpretation to do their job effectively. Every manager's performance now has a financial dimension and their own performance will be judged, at least in part, in the context of the organization's financial record.

These managers are one important group for whom this book has been produced, whether they have experience through long service within the NHS or have transferred into the NHS from the private sector. Just as those who are well versed in the traditional NHS procedures have to learn aspects of the private sector approach, so those bringing private sector skills have to appreciate that they cannot be implanted into the NHS without modification. The book is not an accounting manual, but, to the extent that performance is judged in financial terms, the accounting links between resource generation and consumption and their representation in financial reports are explained. It assumes that readers have limited financial training, but are keen to develop their financial management skills.

Another group of readers are those who work in NHS finance departments and who now have to come to terms with the new financial environment. For them, much of the terminology and underlying logic owes more to the private sector with which they are not familiar if they have been trained and developed their skills in the public sector. It is also important for those who work in health care purchasers to be aware of the financial management structure of the providers from whom they obtain care on behalf of the populations which they serve.

Any members of the general public not directly employed by, but with an interest in, the NHS are a third group who will also find the book useful. For example, local politicians, journalists, potential NHS managers, those undertaking research and students following courses on the NHS will find the material useful in gaining a fuller understanding of what may appear on the face of it to be a somewhat complex situation.

Two final groups who will find the material covered of particular interest are executive and non-executive directors of health authorities and NHS trusts and general practitioners, whether fundholding or not.

The book is written primarily with an NHS trust in mind. The trusts represent the most complex of the new approach's financial structures and mark a significant departure from the financial management of old NHS units. Where the financial arrangements for directly managed units (DMUs) differ significantly from those for trusts, the differences are clearly identified and explained. Care delivery organizations (hospitals) are also concentrated upon for the same reason.

The management process within the NHS has developed throughout its life, with a marked acceleration in recent years. By studying this development, it is possible to appreciate the pressures and influences which have brought about the present position. At the same time, the way in which the NHS is organized and the funds provided by government are converted into delivered health care need to be understood because these provide the financial environment within which the financial management structures have to operate. The first two chapters provide introductory information to explain the development of financial management in the NHS and fill in the background against which it has to be conducted. Chapter 1 describes what financial management is, traces its development and explains the connection between the consumption of resources and the financial consequences. Chapter 2 deals with the structure and funding of the NHS, its constituent parts, and how they are interrelated.

At the present time, the NHS is undergoing the most fundamental reform since it was created. A consequence of this is that procedures are still changing, and they will continue to change. However, these changes are more in the detail than the substance of how it is structured and managed, and so the principles given in this book remain applicable. The reader must be aware of the continuing evolution which is taking place, and, if up-to-date knowledge is needed, for example when deciding what information to provide in an application for trust status, then the appropriate internal documents must be consulted.

Financial information comes in two forms depending upon the user. The first type of financial information is represented by the financial reports that are provided for users external to the organization. These reports are the formal financial accounts, and an insight into how they are prepared and what they mean is presented in Chapters 3, 4 and 5. Chapter 3 deals with cash flows and shows how they arise; this is particularly important as all decisions have cash consequences and the organization as a whole has to operate subject to a cash limit. Chapter 4 reviews the main accounting reports – the income and expenditure account, the balance sheet and the cash flow statement – and includes a worked example to show how these reports are related. Chapter 5 shows how to use the techniques and reports from Chapters 3 and 4 to achieve control of resources and review the organization's progress and position.

The second type of financial information is that prepared for internal use. It is aimed at managers within the organization to assist in the planning and control of income and expenditure. The techniques of costing, budgeting and pricing are presented in Chapters 6 to 11. It is important to know the costs of different activities undertaken by the providers of health care so that realistic prices can be set; Chapters 6 and 7 explain what costs are, how they behave and how they are recorded. Budgets are used in the NHS to control actual activity, and Chapters 8 and 9 deal with the theory and practice of budgeting. Chapters 10 and 11 bring together the techniques of costing and budgeting to develop the method by which prices are derived for negotiation between purchasers and providers.

The final four chapters deal with some specific issues. Chapter 12 examines how contracts between purchasers and providers are negotiated and subsequently controlled. Chapter 13 outlines how an information system can be operated to capture the multitude of individual transactions and events which take place in a facility, analyse and summarize them, and finally report them in a meaningful way. The scale of the NHS makes detailed central control impossible, and it is a stated aim of the government to give as much local autonomy as possible. This desire has to be balanced against the need for the NHS as a whole to function in accordance with central policy, and Chapter 14 explains the ways in which the required regulation is achieved. The final chapter, Chapter 15, draws together the main strands of the book, and considers likely future developments.

Questions are included at the ends of chapters. Solutions are provided for a number of questions as indicated by an asterisk, but others are left for open-ended consideration and, possibly, discussion. A bibliography is also included for those readers who may wish to pursue particular topics to greater depth, as is a list of common abbreviations and acronyms.

The objective is to provide an insight into the new world of financial management in the NHS since *Working for Patients*. The book provides material of interest to everyone concerned with the workings of the NHS and the pressures and constraints under which it has to function. In particular, we feel that effective managers should know how the techniques of financial management can be used to make better decisions. Better decisions mean better management, and therefore lead to an optimization of the manner in which the finite resources provided to the NHS are used. This in turn leads to better patient care, which is the ultimate aim of all those concerned with, or involved in, the activities of the modern National Health Service.

We would like to thank Alan Nelson of Chapman & Hall and Professor John Perrin for their help and encouragement.

HM
NM
SH

Cardiff
17 March 1993

List of abbreviations

ABC	activity-based costing
ACCA	Association of Chartered Certified Accountants
ALOS	average length of stay
AVCO	average cost (of stock)
BACS	Bankers Automatic Clearing Service
BTS	Blood Transfusion Service
CBA	cost−benefit analysis
CCAB	Consultative Committee of Accountancy Bodies
CCE	completed consultant episodes
CCT	compulsory competitive tendering
CCU	coronary care unit
CD	clinical directorate or clinical director
CEO	chief executive officer
CHAAP	Community Health Activity Analysis Package
CHC	Community Health Council
CIMA	Chartered Institute of Management Accountants
CIP	cost improvement programme
CIPFA	Chartered Institute of Public Finance and Accountancy
CLMS	clinical management system
CMB	clinical management budget
CMM	case mix management
CMS	contract management system
CoManDS	Contract Management and Decision Support System
CSSD	central sterile supplies department
D&D	deaths and discharges
DCF	discounted cash flow
DGH	district general hospital
DGM	district general manager
DHA	district health authority

DHSS	Department of Health and Social Services
DMS	director of medical services
DMU	directly managed unit
DoF	director of finance
DoH	Department of Health
DoN	director of nursing
DRG	diagnosis related group
DSS	Department of Social Services
ECR	extra contractual referral
EES	employee's NI contribution
EFL	external financing limit
ERS	employer's NI and superannuation contribution
FCE	finished consultant episodes
FCS	financial control system
FHSA	Family Health Services Authority
FIFO	first in first out – stock valuation
FIS	financial information system
FRS	Financial Reporting Standard
GDP	Gross Domestic Product
GP	general practitioner
GPFH	general practitioner fundholder
HFMA	Healthcare Financial Management Association
HISS	hospital information support system
HMSO	Her Majesty's Stationery Office
HSPI	Health Service Price Index
I&E	income and expenditure
IBD	interest bearing debt
ICAEW	Institute of Chartered Accountants in England and Wales
IRIS	Interactive Resource Information System
IT	information technology
ITU	intensive therapy unit
LIFO	last in first out – stock valuation
MPE	manpower equivalent
MRI	magnetic resonance imager
NAHAT	National Association of Health Authorities and Trusts
NCR	non-contractual referral
NHS	National Health Service
NHSME	National Health Service Management Executive
NHST	National Health Service Trust
NI	National Insurance (contribution)
NPV	net present value

voiced since the 1974 reorganization and probably even before that. However, they have shown a marked increase in number and volume from the mid 1980s onwards and it is apparent that this is now, rightly or wrongly, the perception of the general public. This perception is always likely to remain no matter what level of funding is provided or whichever political party is in power. As funding rises so too do the expectations.

Underfunding accusations are, not unexpectedly, refuted by the government as frequently as they are voiced by others. What cannot be refuted is that the demand for health care exceeds the amount that is being made available by the current pattern of resource provision and consumption. This could mean, at either of two extremes, that:

- the current pattern of resource provision and consumption is absolutely correct, in which case more resources (and hence funding) are needed, or
- the funding level is absolutely correct but an inappropriate mix of resources are being provided and consumed, i.e. they are not being put to best use.

The truth lies somewhere in between, but the problem is knowing exactly where. Even some ardent champions of the underfunding cause demonstrate a recognition of this fact, perhaps unknowingly, when they support their contentions with the allegation that too much money is being spent in certain areas (usually administration) to the detriment of others (usually nursing). The correct answer is not easy to find, as shown by the fact that no one has yet been able to establish categorically and irrefutably how much should be spent. What is certain is that an answer cannot be found without:

- gaining a detailed understanding of existing resource provision and consumption patterns;
- examining whether net improvements to the volume and/or quality of health care are possible by adjusting such patterns;
- implementing the changes necessary to bring about such adjustments.

All of this is an integral part of proper resource management because, as discussed above, resource management – and hence financial management – is concerned not just with what has been, is being and will be spent, but whether it could have been, can be and could be better spent. Financial management is a key tool in determining both the correct distribution of and the correct volume of funding.

Identifying resources

There are at least two important aspects to any resource:

- how much is available and obtainable – quantity;
- how good it is for the intended purpose – quality.

Resources in the National Health Service, as is the case with any commercial concern, cover far more than simply the finance available, and can be classified under four main headings.

Staff

This resource comprises the individual employees and groups of employees essential to the provision of health care. These form a major part of revenue spending within the NHS, being as high as 80% of total costs. The overall value of this resource is reflected not only in terms of numbers of staff (i.e. quantity), but also in terms of their ability, competence and experience, which are generally taken as indicators of quality. As any supervisor or manager of staff can confirm, it is primarily quality rather than quantity of staff that is of importance.

Assets, facilities and consumables

This includes all tangible and intangible assets, equipment, furnishings, consumables, etc., and all services not supplied directly by NHS staff, for example external catering contracts.

These resources can be divided into two further major sub-headings.

- **Revenue** items and services generally are those which are expected to be fully consumed in a relatively short time after acquisition (less than one year). Some are purchased and held as stock with the stock being drawn on as required, for example provisions, drugs and dressings, stationery and heating oil. For other items acquisition automatically equates to consumption, for example most services and utilities such as gas, electricity and telephones.
- **Capital** items generally have an anticipated life-span of more than one year, and can range from general equipment having an expected life of just a few years, through major medical equipment and plant having a life of one or many decades, to freehold land having an indefinite life. Whilst these items normally tend to be tangible, they can also include intangible items such as patents and licences.

Once again it is the mix of quality and quantity available that is important to the proper delivery of health care. Interestingly, this does not always appear to be a generally accepted notion. When it comes to the possibility of hospital closures with service transfers to newer and more modern buildings, the emotive issue of concern to the general public, and even to some NHS staff, is that of quantity rather than quality.

Information and information systems

This resource can also be broken down into two major sub-headings.

- **Information** should not be confused with raw data. Information differs from data in that it represents facts or figures provided in such a way that they are both meaningful and useful in assisting the recipient to perform a defined function. This implies accuracy, relevance, appropriateness and timeliness of delivery. The emphasis is heavily on the quality of information and not its volume or quantity. Indeed too great a volume of information can be detrimental rather than beneficial, as too much can lead to confusion rather than enlightenment.

- **Information systems** are the channels via which information is collected, collated and distributed to those who require access to it. Information systems are a process that involves the generation, transmission, manipulation and evaluation of information. The process should not be confused with the specific tools used in the process, such as computers, telephones or written reports. In other words, information systems can be described as channels of communication – the infrastructure by which information is received and transmitted both internally and externally.

The formal and informal channels of information communication within, for example, a hospital will have been built up over many years and developed to suit changing information requirements as they arise. High quality information and information systems are essential. Unfortunately, being perhaps the least tangible of resources, information and information systems are very often forgotten altogether or are considered low priority, particularly in times of organizational change and financial stringency. Such an oversight or opinion misses an important point: information, as defined above, and the channels for communicating it correctly and accurately should be seen as integral parts of resource management, and hence financial management.

Finance

This not only facilitates the acquisition of other resources but, given the huge diversity of individual resources required to provide modern health care, also provides a common means of measuring and valuing such diverse consumption. All resource use is expressed in the common language of money. It is a language which managers from all disciplines understand. There is no concept of quality of this resource, only quantity! If resources, and hence finance, are to be managed, a value, expressed in financial terms, must be placed upon the consumption of a resource over a period.

Choice and the challenge of resource management

There are many difficulties and challenges facing all those responsible for the provision of health care at all levels in the NHS. Perhaps the single greatest challenge is the fact that choices have to be made. This can be expressed as the requirement by those managing the delivery of modern health care to provide optimum answers to certain key questions, namely:

- What services will be provided?
- How much of these services will be provided?
- Where will these services be provided?
- How will these services be provided?

Strategically, for example, choices have to be made as to: numbers of hospitals, clinics and health centres, and their physical locations; the specialties and services to be made available; and the types and planned level of treatments. Operationally, similar discussions take place at various levels within the NHS. In all such instances formal managerial mechanisms are used, whereby explicit decisions are taken after weighing up the perceived costs and benefits of the alternatives.

The cut-off point of such formal managerial decisions is normally where it concerns an individual patient rather than patients as a group. Below that level, choices need to be made not only between treatment regimes for individual patients, but between patients and between length and quality of life. Such choices are made by clinical staff.

When an explicit decision is taken at any level to follow one course of action, and thereby consume limited resources in a particular manner, effectively this is an implicit decision not to take any of the alternative courses that could have been followed with that same funding. This applies to every spending decision, from the size and location of a hospital, through the number and grade mix of staff, to the treatment regime applied to a patient. However, it also applies in a more fundamental way. Assume a life-extending treatment for a young child costs £20 000 and a hip operation for an elderly patient costs £1000. An explicit decision to treat a child at that cost is also an implicit decision not to spend that same money on providing 20 hip operations, assuming waiting lists exist for such operations. Within the total funding limit, money may be made available to undertake a certain amount of both types of intervention, but there must come a point when the 'final' £20 000 is reached. At that point, assuming unsatisfied demand for both types of intervention, a decision as to whether to spend the £20 000 one way of the other has to be taken.

Given their importance, decisions concerned with the availability and distribution of health care at all levels should be well-informed and explicit. One of the challenges of resource management, at all levels, is therefore recognizing, appreciating and accepting the potential advantages of a more explicit consideration of the relative benefits arising from different ways of consuming the same resource – in other words, arriving at a position whereby you know the best way to spend your next £ and your final £.

Information is needed about both the costs and benefits of all the alternatives before a proper decision can be made; this is commonly referred to as evaluating the 'input–output equation'. Whilst the measurement and valuation of resource consumption, the inputs, is relatively straightforward, this is not the case with the measurement and valuation of the ultimate benefit, the outputs. This difficulty arises from the fact that there is an inherent problem in attempting even to measure, let alone value, the benefit of the NHS, which ultimately is an improvement in the health status of the population. On the input, or costs, side there are similar, but less fundamental, problems in attempting accurately to link resource consumption to individual patients or groups of patients.

Systems supporting the process of resource management ideally should provide management, clinicians and finance staff with a single integrated set of data from which to extract information for use in the decision-making process. It is apparent that an enormous amount of work has to be undertaken before such systems can be relied upon totally. Therefore, recognizing that there will inevitably be shortcomings, an identification, acknowledgement and acceptance of, and preferably contribution towards, the principles upon which these systems are constructed will at least allow users to come to terms with the situation and to accept them with all their shortcomings. Gaining this understanding and appreciation of the principles is therefore a further major challenge.

Linked to an understanding of principles is the need to gain a fuller picture of the entire process of health care provision. Problems arise when resource managers understand only part of the extremely complex process, perhaps only the part in which they directly are involved. The view of such managers can be too narrow when wider issues are discussed.

The challenge of making decisions is heightened by the fact that less than adequate information is available, even though theory dictates that the receipt of adequate information is a key requirement if consistently sensible decisions are to be taken. In practice the best use has to be made of what is available. To do this, information is needed about what can be provided and how it can be obtained. By comparing this with the ideal, it is possible to identify how the situation can be improved.

The nature of the NHS means that functioning within an explicit decision-making process often makes things much harder rather than easier. Perhaps this at least partially explains why, despite the best efforts of health economists, traditionally within the NHS so many fundamental decisions have been taken implicitly, and are either poorly informed or uninformed in the two key areas of cost and benefit. The introduction of contracting arrangements in 1991 started to change this fairly dramatically, and the formal contracting process is in itself designed to ensure that the fundamental resource distribution decision-making process is now far more explicit and better informed, with the intent that this leads to improved resource distribution and utilization, leading in turn to a higher level of health care provision.

When first introduced, these new arrangements proved immensely unpopular with many clinical staff. It was felt – and by some is still felt – unethical to adopt an explicit process whereby numbers of patients to be treated in each of a mix of specialties should be specified. Yet the contra argument is that if the historical distribution of resources and hence delivery of health care is proved not to produce optimum benefit, then is it not unethical to continue such a distribution?

In summary, the role of those managing resources within the NHS is to control the process by which health benefit is obtained with the intent of optimizing this benefit. This would not be an easy task even in a perfect world and is made infinitely more arduous by the difficulty in obtaining accurate costs of resource consumption decisions at a useful level coupled with the current incapability to measure and value the true final output of the NHS.

Value for money

Reflecting the increasing importance placed upon the efficient and effective use of limited resources, central government continues to place greater and greater emphasis upon the search for value for money (VFM) in all public services. Value for money is, in essence, a cost–benefit analysis, involving a joint consideration of resources consumed and value obtained. VFM initiatives come in many shapes and sizes and have been with us for many years. The annual cost improvement programme (CIP) is one manifestation, as are such things as secondary income targets, compulsory competitive tendering (CCT), high level performance indicators and annual review mechanisms.

Included within the financial projections, commonly called proformas, produced by each trust is a section identifying anticipated patient volumes. This is also the case with, indeed the purpose of, purchasers' health plans. The production of such detail allows central government to examine activity levels in the context of associated costs. More recently, the introduction of annual contract productivity increases, whereby perhaps 1% or 2% extra work is undertaken for no additional contract income, continues the quest. So to does benchmarking, which encourages managers continually to measure performance against the acknowledged 'best' in each area and to identify, implement and test processes that aim to beat the best.

Each of these schemes, initiatives and impositions is designed to ensure that managers at all levels within the service give consideration to the relationships between costs and benefits leading to an identification and exploration of areas where improvements could potentially be made. Integral to VFM is an identification of relevant considerations that can get ignored, or are allocated a low priority, under the more technical evaluations of efficiency and effectiveness. Quality issues are normally the most important of these, although often where quality standards are specified their level of achievement becomes a part of the measure of effectiveness.

VFM units have been established to aid this process. Their role includes identifying best practice and assisting in the development of specific VFM schemes. Where particular schemes demonstrate a suitable degree of success normally they are publicized in sufficient detail with the intent that they be adopted or adapted for use by others.

However, perhaps the greatest incentive for increased value for money within the service has been the introduction of contracting arrangements. Market forces in the private sector are considered to be a stimulus for ensuring that a range of 'value for money' products and services are available in practically all markets. The introduction of contracting to the NHS and the encouragement of a form of competition between providers is clearly intended to bring such forces to bear within the public health sector in the belief that this will dramatically increase the value for money obtained from available resources.

A history of financial management in the NHS

Prior to 1974, financial management was limited to the control of costs on what is termed a 'subjective' basis, that is by the type of staff employed and goods/services purchased. The focus was on the identification of 'on what' the money was spent. Budgeting was at its most basic, with simple roll-over historical budgets and no clear definition of lines of financial management or responsibility. The 1974 NHS reorganization swept this away, clearly placing the emphasis on organization, and hence management, using a 'functional' basis. This placed an increased emphasis on the need to identify where the money was being spent. That fundamental revision has had far reaching effects for Health Service financial management but it was not until a decade and half later that a widespread move away from financial management on a purely functional basis could be accomplished with any degree of confidence.

The 1982 reorganization effectively pushed the authority and accountability for resource consumption decisions to the unit level, this being seen as an essential complement to the new unit management arrangements. Maximum delegation of budget responsibility down to and within units was encouraged, but the emphasis was still firmly on the functional approach. That still left the basic problem that those responsible for taking the day-to-day organizational decisions that determined patterns and volumes of resource consumption were not responsible for the budgets bearing the costs and hence managerially or financially accountable for their actions.

This problem had been recognized. Even by the time of the 1982 reorganization a great deal of work had been undertaken to tackle the first stage of the solution, namely identifying costs on a 'clinical' basis, that is relating them to the 'outputs' – or more accurately 'throughputs' – of the service, rather than to the 'inputs'. Included under this head were alternative, but generally complementary, approaches to costing by clinician, by groups or 'firms' of clinicians, by patient, by disease and by specialty. However, it is felt by many commentators that it was the needs of the Health Service planners, with their particular interest in optimization of health care resource utilization between types and location for very large patient groups, that decided matters in favour of costing by specialty – or, as it formally became known, 'specialty costing'.

In 1980 a DHSS Steering Group, chaired by Mrs Edith Körner, was set up to review and report on the financial information available in the NHS, with particular reference to:

- its suitability to the management requirements of the NHS;
- its quality;
- the degree to which input measures, as expressed in financial performance infor- mation, were being, and could better be, matched against 'output' measures – or more accurately the activity performance measures which were deemed to act as proxy indicators.

The 'Körner Report', as it became known, made a number of important recom- mendations, amongst which were:

- The existing subjective analysis of expenditure should be retained.
- Costs should be identified by 'site', a term which had already been defined for existing cost returns, and by department/function within site. This represented an extension of the existing detailed functional analysis into what often is termed cost-centre analysis.
- Activity/workload measures should be developed for each department/function appropriate to their particular 'output', as measured by their throughput. This would allow the development of functional efficiency measures.
- To improve management and planning information, functional costs should also be matched against clinical activity. Whilst costs could be apportioned over such activity in a number of different ways, the most appropriate, given the current development of techniques, was to adopt the relatively tried and tested specialty costing approach.
- Such apportionments should be undertaken on the basis of the activity/workload information already recommended for collection.

It did not advise specifically on whether clinicians should be involved in the management of resources by becoming budget holders, and the emphasis was on costing rather than on budgeting. The Report also concluded that, due to the lack of consideration of case mix, specialty costing could only be a step on the way to clinical costing and subsequently clinical budgeting.

Up to this point it is apparent that the general emphasis had continued to be on functional budgeting. The widely recognized problem was that this approach did not provide budgets that matched information on inputs, as measured by resource consumption and hence cost, directly with information on final outputs, measured as throughputs. Nor did it always place the responsibility for the control of that element of resource consumption affected by the type and volume of final outputs in the hands of those best in a position to exercise such control, namely the clinicians.

The costing techniques available to reallocate functional costs against clinical activity served both to emphasize the value of such costing information for financial and operational planning purposes, and to demonstrate the difficulties faced in its ongoing derivation to an acceptable level of accuracy and reliability. Certainly, the level of accuracy and reliability acceptable for costing purposes was recognized as inadequate for clinically based budgeting, given the existing financial management arrangements in the NHS.

The Griffiths Inquiry Report on NHS Management, published in late 1983, contained a number of wide-ranging recommendations, the majority of which are linked to the major recommendation of a move from functional management to general management. Integral with such a move was the further delegation of accountability for budget performance to unit level.

The Report highlighted the fact that the current functional approach to budgeting was, in effect, nothing more than a means by which spending limits were allocated to budget managers and actual spending performance against these limits was recorded and compared. Generally there was neither reference to activity levels of any type, even functional/departmental activity or workload measures, which meant a lack of ongoing assessment of functional/departmental efficiency, nor any involvement of clinical staff in financial issues. For general management to prove dynamic and responsive to the changing environment, the monitoring of financial performance had to cease simply being the passive consideration of sets of figures and had to become an integral and active part of management's measurement and evaluation of organizational efficiency and effectiveness. This new approach to the management of resources was identified by the generic title **management budgeting**.

Management budgeting involved a recognition of the value to the organization, both strategically and operationally, of financial information as a management tool contributing to overall performance monitoring, rather than as a target spending limit. Although not by any means a new idea, the greater involvement of clinicians in this resource management and control process was seen not only as an essential development, but also as a logical one. It was suggested that this involvement should take the form of clinicians becoming budget holders/managers and hence managers of resources. At that time it was anticipated that the natural end-point was for budgets to be held by individual clinicians and reflect all costs attributable to their clinical activity. Some commentators therefore, perhaps more correctly, use the term 'clinical management budgeting' when referring to the Griffiths recommendation.

This development involved fundamental changes to the financial management arrangements in the NHS and, at least in theory, appeared to be the step forward required to introduce clinicians both to general management and to financial management. Four demonstration sites were selected to undertake an implementation of the management budgeting proposals. However, management budgeting was not successful.

Its successor, the formal Resource Management Initiative (RMI) was announced in Health Notice (86)34. As with its predecessor the emphasis was placed on developing, in conjunction with clinical staff, local management processes for planning and controlling the use of resources. There were, however, a few subtle but important differences. In particular, the emphasis was on the involvement of medical and nursing staff as partners in the project. General managers were expected to set as their most important and declared objective their building of the RMI upon the foundation of the commitment to the NHS of such staff. Most importantly, general and medical managers alike were required to view financial management as playing a supporting rather than a leading role, albeit a highly important one.

Six hospital and eleven community sites were selected for demonstration RMI projects over the period 1986–1988. There was no central instruction as to the management structures to be adopted at these sites, nor as to specific information systems or infrastructures to be used. The intention was that by leaving the development of such matters to local discretion alternative approaches would inevitably evolve and, from both failure and success, useful lessons could be learned.

In the spring of 1989 it was announced that the RMI had become official policy and that it would be 'rolled out' to a further 50 hospital sites, with the eventual aim of implementation in all 280 large acute hospitals in England. A number of early lessons were learned from the initial demonstration and roll-out sites.

First, it became apparent that the key to successful implementation lay in determining the local management structure most appropriate to the particular operational needs of the unit, and then designing and implementing the supporting resource information systems around this structure. The alternative approach of forcing management structures to fit predetermined information system designs reduced the perceived degree of success.

As part of the development of the necessary management arrangements, structures based on clinical directorates started to emerge, involving clinicians not only in the day-to-day budget management process but also in operational and strategic planning. The emphasis was on the involvement of clinicians as groups or firms, with each group having a designated clinical director responsible for the directorate's budget performance. This contrasted with the management budgeting approach of individual clinicians managing their own budgets.

This development recognized that involvement in resource management inevitably requires involvement in general management, and the clinical directorate concept fits neatly into the Griffiths general management proposals. The opposite is equally true as involvement in general management inevitably requires involvement in resource management.

Secondly, whilst the information systems implemented in the demonstration sites generally were quite different, the common factor in each was the identification of costs at patient level and the allocation of these costs to individual patients. This patient-centred approach was recognized as essential for providing to general and clinical managers key financial information required for the resource utilization decision process. This approach has subsequently manifested itself in the guise of information systems known by the generic term **case mix management**. By late 1991 each of the 280 English acute sites had commenced the project to some degree or other, with the early sites entering the final phases of the implementation.

The goal of resource management can be defined as being to improve the effectiveness of resource use, and to improve the quantity and quality of health care available. In practical terms this has been expressed in the aim of providing management, clinicians and finance staff with a single integrated set of data on which to base decisions. Thus, in general terms, its aim is to provide managers at all levels with the information to make informed decisions.

At the time of writing it is impossible to comment as to whether the RMI has achieved its goal nationally, simply because implementation to the planned stage of development will not be completed at the vast majority of sites for many years. However, at the commission of the Department of Health, an independent evaluation of the six initial pilot sites has been undertaken by a group of researchers at Brunel University. This commenced in May 1988 and took the form of a structured analysis of costs and benefits. The group's final report was published in mid 1991, and prompted some fierce debate. Critics of the RMI point to the comments in the report that state there have been no measurable additional benefits to patient care, measured by increases in effectiveness, nor any release of funds giving an increase in efficiency. Supporters of RMI point to the indisputable fact that, in the absence of clearly defined measures and valuations of health status, a cost–benefit analysis concentrating primarily upon such outcomes gives too little weight to other types of benefit, whether measurable or perceived. Certainly, in response to the report, senior staff involved with the RMI at the pilot sites felt that it had omitted to identify a range of benefits, both tangible and intangible, from improved financial management of budgets through to the more esoteric 'cultural change'. The overall conclusion can perhaps only be seen as inconclusive, a view echoed by the group themselves when they stated that four years after the announcement of the RMI, they were still unable to provide a definite assessment of RM as an ongoing working process for hospital management.

The creation of the post-reforms 'market-place' was assumed by some commentators at the time, albeit briefly, as meaning the end of the formal RMI. Such a view overlooked the fact that the RMI has always been intended to be a means to an end and not an end in itself. The RMI is a multifunction management tool designed specifically to assist in the achievement of a stated goal, that of optimization of health gain and health status, by encouraging the efficient use of resources through planning spending patterns and comparing actual outcome to these plans. The main change arising from the introduction of contracting and the market-centred environment is the level, type and source of pressures forcing efficient resource use and hence that achievement.

Not surprisingly, it was rapidly realized that the contracting environment has actually increased the need for the RMI or an equivalent process. There is now little doubt that the RMI, which was gaining increasing acceptance as useful under the previously simplistic approach to funding, is now seen as essential under the more sophisticated contracting approach. Indeed, the RMI could flourish under practically any approach to funding, but the contracting approach to funding would not long survive without either the RMI or something conceptually similar.

Conclusion

Good financial management in the NHS stems from effective and efficient resource use. Developing a culture capable of supporting a suitable system of financial management has proved to be a lengthy process with success coming in small stages. The government reforms of the early 1990s represented a fundamental reshaping of the organizational and financial structure of the NHS. Since that time, the benefit of gaining skills in financial management by all those involved in the NHS has become of ever increasing value.

Questions

1. What is meant by the term 'financial management'? Describe its development within the NHS.
2. What are the main types of resources which the NHS uses in the process of delivering health care?
3. Differentiate between resource management and financial management and explain the extent to which they are interlinked.
4. To what extent does the NHS have an explicit decision-making apparatus. Does the existence of an explicit decision-making regime make the process of decision taking harder or easier than using an implicit one?
5. The fundamental questions facing the NHS are fairly easy to identify:

   - What services should be provided?
   - How much of these services should be provided?
   - Where will these services be provided?
   - How will these services be provided?

   Answering all of these questions, in practice, means choosing between alternative courses of action. What problems arise when making those choices?
6. 'Financial management means trying to find ways of cutting budgets.' 'Financial management means checking that budgets are not overspent.' To what extent, if at all, are these two statements true? With what is financial management concerned?
7. 'Choices about the provision of health care should always be explicit.' Discuss, and defend or dispute.
8. Any assessment of efficiency and/or effectiveness requires a knowledge of outputs. What is the final output of the NHS, and why is it so difficult to measure and value?
9. To what extent has the introduction of the financial management initiatives, such as the formal Resource Management Initiative, changed attitudes of clinicians to management and management to clinicians?
10. In what way can information and information systems be considered a resource? Why is no financial value placed upon them?

2

An outline of the NHS

AIMS

Since its creation in 1948, the objective of the NHS has been to secure an improvement in the health of the population. It does this by providing a comprehensive range of health care which is, with a few exceptions, free of charge at the point of delivery. The service created to meet the objectives is very large and complex, and the functions of its individual parts, and sections within these parts, are best understood if they can be placed against the background of the organization as a whole. It is also useful to have an appreciation of how the NHS is funded and how, in the presence of essentially limitless demand, these funds are converted into specific services for patients. The aims of this chapter are to:

- outline the organizational structure of the NHS as a whole;
- describe the various parts of the NHS and how they fit into its structure;
- describe the flows of funds into and within the NHS;
- explain the operation of the internal market which is used to match health needs with health care delivery;
- outline how financial planning and control is exercised within the NHS.

Organization

The structure of the NHS, as it operates in England, is illustrated in Figure 2.1.

The structure of the NHS is designed to provide a national framework of objectives and priorities which local management is then left to achieve, subject to accountability. The roles of each of the separate parts shown in Figure 2.1 and how they interrelate to each other are as follows:

- **The Department of Health (DoH)** is headed by the Secretary of State for Health who sits in the Cabinet and is responsible to Parliament for the operation of the NHS as a whole.
- **The NHS Policy Board** is chaired by the Secretary of State and is responsible for the development of the strategy which the NHS is to follow in the light of

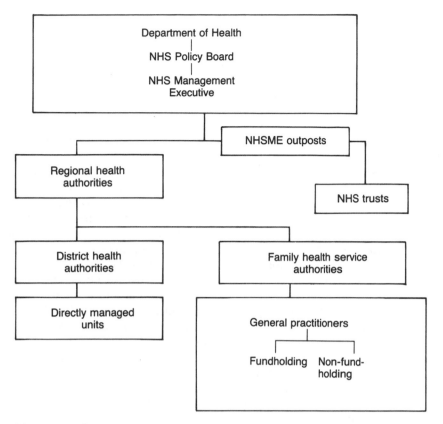

Figure 2.1 The structure of the NHS.

government policy. It sets the objectives of the Management Executive and
monitors the extent of their achievement.
- **The NHS Management Executive (NHSME)** is chaired by a chief executive
and is responsible for putting the strategy, once developed, into operation. It is
accountable to the Policy Board for the management of the NHS.
- **Regional health authorities (RHAs)** have to ensure that government health
policy is carried out within their geographical regions. They set and monitor
performance criteria and provide the framework for the financial planning process
of their subordinate districts, units and FHSAs. When the plans have been
received, they are reviewed to ensure that they are viable and then consolidated
with the RHA plan to provide an aggregate view. The widespread introduction of
trusts eventually led to a review of the role of RHAs, with their responsibilities
being revised to reflect the refocusing of their contribution to the process of
providing health care. They were slimmed down to about one-third of their size
in line with their new prime role of developing effective purchasing, but were not
reduced in number.
- **District health authorities (DHAs)** are responsible for ensuring that the health
needs of the populations which they serve are met. They have to ensure that
there are effective services to prevent and control diseases and promote health.
Where they continue to control management units, they have to set their targets

and monitor performance. The district prepares a financial plan covering its own operations and those of its directly managed units. The development of health care procurement has seen the merging of DHAs to form commissioning agencies, sometimes in conjunction with family health service authorities, or their collaboration to form purchasing consortia.

- **Directly managed units (DMUs)** are hospitals and other health care provider units, such as community care, which have remained under district control as opposed to becoming NHS trusts. Although they are part of the DHA, and their financial results are included in those of the DHA for the purposes of annual accounts, they are effectively separate, self-managing, entities.
- **NHS trusts (NHSTs)** are separate legal entities which, although they are self-governing, remain part of the NHS. The management of each trust is carried out by a board of directors, with a chairman appointed by the Secretary of State. Each board has a number of non-executive directors; their appointment is approved by the Secretary of State in consultation with the chairman, and they are chosen for the contribution it is considered they can make to the effective management of the trust. There are also executive directors who are responsible for putting the board's decisions into operation; these must include a chief executive officer, a medical director, a senior nurse professional and a finance director. When first established, trusts were responsible directly to the NHSME; **NHSME outposts**, which are regionally based, were subsequently introduced.
- **Family health service authorities (FHSAs)** each have 11 members, with a chairman appointed by the Secretary of State and a general manager who is responsible for running the FHSA and implementing policy. Their task is to plan and manage the Family Practitioner Services, which includes overseeing GP practice budgets, indicative prescribing budgets and medical audit. They are funded by their RHA, which is responsible for monitoring and coordinating their plans and reviewing their performance.
- **General practitioners (GPs)** are self-employed, usually functioning in the form of partnerships. They contract with the NHS to provide services to patients, subject to agreed standards, and are overseen by the FHSAs.
- **Fundholding GPs (GPFHs)** receive funds from their RHA based on the number of patients on their registered list. They use these funds to pay for a specified range of treatment required by their patients. A practice is allowed to overspend its budget by up to 5% in a year as long as there are clinical reasons; the excess expenditure is then recouped in the following year. Persistent overspending results in an audit being undertaken, with the possibility of fundholder status being removed from the practice.
- **Non-fundholding GPs** have exactly the same functions and responsibilities towards their patients as fundholders, but the treatment required by their patients is paid for by the DHA from funds provided for this purpose.

Community health councils (CHCs) are not included in Figure 2.1. They are local bodies intended to represent the views of the consumers of the services provided by the NHS. This is achieved by contributing ideas on how the service should be operated and developed, commenting on planned developments and monitoring public satisfaction.

The above outline of the NHS relates to its organization in England; the main structure is the same in other parts of the United Kingdom, but there are some differences:

- **Wales** has no RHA, and so its functions have to be carried out elsewhere. Overall planning, resource allocation and funding of regional services are the responsibility of the NHS Directorate of the Welsh Office. There is a Health Policy Board, chaired by the Secretary of State for Wales, to provide strategic direction, the decisions of which are put into effect by an executive committee of the board headed by the director of the NHS in Wales. Some RHA functions are undertaken by DHAs, while others are the responsibility of the Welsh Health Common Services Authority.
- **Northern Ireland** is organized in a similar way to Wales, but has health and social services boards rather than DHAs. There has been a slower movement towards local management, but this is now being introduced by such measures as the appointment of general managers at major acute hospitals.
- **Scotland** has health boards which are generally similar to the English DHAs, but also run the family practitioner services. There is no separate RHA, and so its responsibilities are shared between the Scottish Office, health boards and a common services organization. The Secretary of State for Scotland is assisted by an advisory council and a chief executive is responsible for putting the overall policy into effect.

Funding in the NHS

The amount of money which is to be spent on the NHS as a whole is set as part of the annual Public Expenditure Survey (PES), and is cash limited, that is spending must not exceed a specified sum. For this to work at the aggregate level, all of the separate parts of the NHS must have strict control of their spending, although it is possible to offset an overspend in one part against an equivalent underspend in another to achieve an overall balance. The funds provided are of two types, revenue and capital. Revenue funds are to be used for the day-to-day running of the service and so pay for such things as salaries and drugs, while capital funds (not to be confused with capital charges) are to acquire new long-life assets such as buildings and equipment. These two types of funds are now considered separately.

Revenue funds

Figure 2.2 shows the flow of revenue funds within the NHS.

The DoH is informed each year of how much it is allowed to spend for revenue purposes. The first call on these funds are certain services which are organized on a national basis, such as heart transplants; these account in total for a relatively small amount of the funds available. It is the intention that, by the mid to late 1990s, the balance of the funds will be distributed to purchasers on the basis of the number of people resident within, or served by, each one, weighted for age and morbidity. This is known as distributing funds on the basis of **weighted capitation**. The DoH also makes adjustments in its allocations to allow for the interest and dividends it receives from NHSTs.

RHAs also receive capital charges, which comprise depreciation and interest, from the DMUs located within their boundaries. These charges do not represent additional

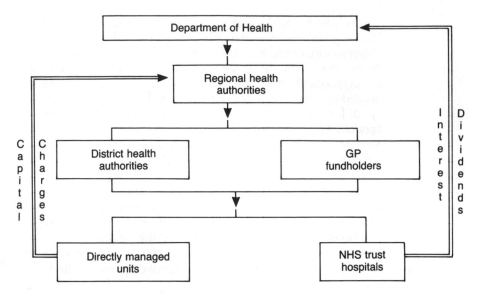

Figure 2.2 Funding the NHS: revenue.

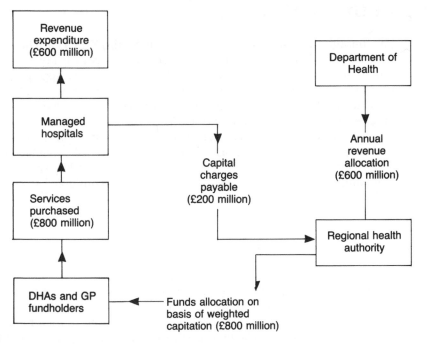

Figure 2.3 Capital charges.

cash as they are added to the funds received from the DoH and redistributed to DHAs; hence they simply flow around within the NHS, as is shown in Figure 2.3. The DoH allocates £600 million to an RHA, which also receives £200 million from the DMUs within its boundaries by way of capital charges. This gives the RHA a total of £800 million to share between the DHAs and GPFHs to buy health care. Payment for the capital charges associated with treatment is included in their payments to DMUs, and this is passed back by the DMUs to the RHA.

The total sum of money available to RHAs, after 'top-slicing' for the costs of running the RHA and providing regional services, is allocated to DHAs and GPFHs. The amount received by each DHA is based on the size of its resident population, less any which are served by a GPFH. GPFHs receive an amount of money based on the number of patients on their list.

Capital funds

Capital funds are divided between RHAs on the basis of weighted population. However, before this is done, the DoH makes an adjustment to allow for capital expenditure undertaken by NHSTs within each region. The NHSTs agree their capital expenditure plans individually with the DoH, and are not funded by the RHA. Therefore, it is only at the level of the DoH that allowance can be made for the amount of capital expenditure undertaken by NHSTs.

Below the RHA, capital funds are distributed on the basis of agreed development plans for large projects, although limited amounts may be allocated downwards to be used at local discretion for small projects.

The internal market

After DHAs and GPFHs have been funded, there is a switch in the distribution process from fund allocation to earning income from contract-based activity. The DHAs and GPFHs, known as 'purchasers', acquire health care on behalf of the population for which they are responsible, and money is said to 'follow the patient' in an internal market. As a result, DMUs and NHSTs, known as providers, receive cash from supplying health care, and the amount of income each can generate is based on the volume of treatment it can deliver. This has been likened to a 'market for health care', but there is an important difference between this and a true market, since the NHS 'market' has to operate subject to a cash limit. In a 'proper' market, excess demand initially gives rise to higher profits which attract additional suppliers until demand is satisfied at a price providing an adequate profit. In a cash limited market, where the accumulation of surpluses is explicitly forbidden, excess demand gives rise to waiting lists.

First we can consider the choices facing the purchasers of health care. This is illustrated in Figure 2.4.

Faced with the choices shown in Figure 2.4, and limited in the amount of money it has available to spend, each DHA has to develop a health procurement plan based on the care required by its residents. In developing this plan, some funds must be held back for contingencies which are likely to arise during the year and to meet the cost of extra contractual referrals. There is no requirement for the DHA to favour its own DMUs, and it should seek to achieve the greatest possible value for money. As a result, facilities offering best value will flourish, while those that are relatively expensive will not attract much income; this acts as an incentive for providers to

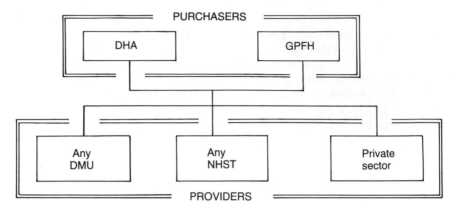

Figure 2.4 Purchasing health care.

increase their efficiency. Where the best value for money is offered by private sector facilities, purchasers are free to use them.

DHAs do not have total freedom on how to spend their funds, as they must ensure that local access to specified core services is guaranteed:

- accident and emergency departments;
- admission to hospital from an accident and emergency department;
- other cases where urgent admission is required;
- out-patient and other support services required by the first three core services;
- other services which have to be provided on a local basis, such as district nursing and services for elderly people.

Once the provision of these core service has been established, DHAs can take a flexible approach to meeting the other requirements of their populations. It is in these areas that the greatest possibility of 'shopping around' to achieve maximum value for money lies.

GPFHs arrange treatment for their patients in respect of a specified group of services and pay for it using funds from the RHA. The services covered are:

- a defined list of in-patient and day case treatments, such as bronchoscopy and tonsillectomy;
- out-patient services;
- diagnostic investigation;
- drugs prescribed and dispensed.

The relatively small size of GPFHs compared with DHAs makes them less able to accommodate large expenditures on individual patients, and, where the cost of such treatment exceeds a centrally specified sum, it becomes the responsibility of the DHA. As well as flexibility in where treatment is purchased, the GPFH also has the ability to switch funds between headings so that, for example, reduced expenditure on drugs can be spent on other treatments.

Turning to the providers within the NHS, the position facing DMUs and NHSTs as regards the sources of their funds is shown in Figure 2.5. This shows that DMUs and NHSTs can derive their patient-related income from a number of separate sources:

- **GPFHs** buy services on behalf of their patients from any source which they consider appropriate.

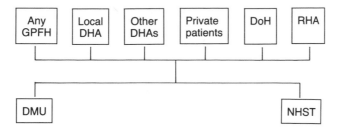

Figure 2.5 Funding DMUs and NHSTs.

- **The local DHA** within which the unit is located buys services for the members of its resident population which are not funded through a GPFH.
- **Other DHAs** are free to buy health care from facilities located outside their boundaries.
- **Private patients** can buy health care, possible through the use of private health care insurance schemes. The amount they pay represents additional income for the NHS.
- **The DoH** can pay for the facility to provide supra-regional services.
- **RHAs** can pay for the facility to provide regional services.

The purchaser/provider interface

The separation between purchasers and providers of health care gives two resource flows which have to be balanced for the service as a whole to keep within its cash limit:

- Purchasers have to ensure that they do not commit themselves to spending more than is received. On the other hand, they do not want to be left with unspent sums at the end of the year as this means that, since there are waiting lists, some of their residents remained untreated when this need not have been so.
- Providers receive virtually all their income from purchasers, and have to ensure that their expenditure does not exceed their income. If they incur deficits, then more resources are being consumed than is allowed by the cash limit, and a surplus implies that the same services could have been supplied at lower prices; this would have left extra funds with the purchasers with which to buy more care.

The relationship between purchasers and providers is regulated by the use of contracts. These can be:

- contracts within the NHS
- management budgets, which are effectively contracts between DHAs and their subordinate DMUs
- contracts with the private sector.

As is the case in the commercial sector, these contracts specify the nature and level of the service to be provided and the basis on which payment is to be made.

There are three types of contract:

- **Block contracts** involve the purchase, for an annual fee, of access to an agreed range of services. These are particularly appropriate for core services where it is necessary to maintain a level of capacity.

  For the purchaser, this type of contract is beneficial as it sets the amount to be paid in advance and so removes uncertainty about costs. However, problems may arise if the actual volume of cases or the mix of cases differs significantly from those predicted when the contracts were entered into. In these circumstances, some of the agreed, and paid for, services may be under-used, while excess demand for others puts unanticipated pressure on the provider.

  Providers, under these contracts, have the advantage of knowing, in advance, that a regular cash flow will be received. On the other hand, they have to carry the risk that a higher case load than expected will arise, or that costs will increase at a rate in excess of that anticipated when the contract was entered into.

  To some extent, the problems for both purchasers and providers can be overcome by including in the contract indicative levels of usage and how cost increases are to be accommodated.

- **Cost and volume contracts** pay providers a sum for the provision of a set level of service, usually expressed as a maximum number of treatments, cases or interventions. Once the agreed maximum is reached, additional payment is made on the basis of individual cases. The contract must specify an overall limit on the number of cases it covers so that the purchasers can maintain control over their expenditure, which cannot be done if an open-ended commitment is made to pay for all instances when a treatment is provided.

  These contracts give the purchaser certainty about the minimum level of its financial commitment, but could cause financial problems if it enters into a number of them and the actual usage of all of them is at or near the maximum contracted activity level. The purchaser is unlikely to have budgeted on the basis that all contracts would operate at their maximum level and so is potentially committed to expenditure in excess of income. In the same way as block contracts, there is also the risk of wasting resources through under-utilization if the number of cases treated is less than the minimum agreed or the cases are less complex than anticipated. The extent of these problems is influenced by both the relative and actual spread between the agreed minimum and the maximum number of cases.

  The provider is given the certainty of a minimum level of funding, but is left with uncertainty about the number of excess referrals, and hence income that will be generated.

- **Cost per case contracts** are used to pay for instances where patients are not covered by either of the other types. For example, a patient may be referred to a specialist unit in another region with which there is no other contractual arrangement. It is also possible to have an agreement with a local provider that particular types of case, up to an agreed limit, will be paid for on an individual basis. The agreement of the purchaser to pay for cost per case treatment must be obtained before the treatment is undertaken.

  The purchaser has to retain uncommitted funds to meet the cost of this type of contract. The amount of funds is likely to be determined by experience, but there is a danger that it will be minimal with the result that the ability to meet *ad hoc* requirements will be limited.

Each purchaser is likely to hold contracts of all three types with a number of providers. In the case of facilities supplying regional and national specialties this could involve a significant number of separate contracts. This means that providers must have in place efficient systems to monitor treatments provided and ensure that they are billed in the appropriate way.

The block contracts and the fixed part of cost and volume contracts given providers a predetermined minimum income. This allows them to plan for a minimum level of service provision. However, it also means that funds are not strictly following the individual patient with the result that the market operates in terms of blocks of provision rather than unique patient episodes. This reduces flexibility, since:

- The purchaser cannot respond quickly to market opportunities and take advantage of lower prices elsewhere. This could only by overcome if every contract was on a cost per case basis, and this is not a practical proposition. A further difference with a true market scenario arises when this aspect is considered. Units within the NHS are not allowed to offer 'cut-price' services to attract patients in specialties where there is competition; this option is open to private sector providers. The rules by which this is enforced:

  - require total income to cover all costs, including the return on capital;
  - do not allow cross-subsidization whereby deficits are allowed on some treatments which are offset by surpluses on others;
  - only allow treatments to be provided at marginal cost where they utilize spare capacity.

- The penalty of withdrawing custom because of poor service cannot be exercised quickly. The response to this is to build performance aims into the contracts to cover such quality issues as waiting times, complaints procedures and acceptable facilities. Medical audit is relied upon to maintain the standard of the care.

The variable part of the cost and volume contracts and the cost per case contracts provide flexibility, especially where there is an element of choice about where and when treatment takes place. In these circumstances, money really does follow the patient. Hospitals able to attract such cases benefit from additional income, while purchasers benefit by obtaining care as cost-effectively as possible.

Where contractual arrangements exist, whether in the NHS or elsewhere, disputes are bound to arise about one or the other party's rights or obligations. As a first step to avoiding disputes, as far as possible, model forms of contract have been developed with the help of the NHSME. Where differences between the parties do arise, mechanisms exist to settle them:

- Arbitration arrangements have been set up to deal with disputes where the contracting parties are both within the NHS but have no direct management relationship.
- Where the contracts take the form of management budgets, as is the case with the relationship between DHAs and their DMUs, they can be operated through the normal means of managerial control.
- Contracts with the private sector are subject to the usual legal means of enforcement and redress.

Non-contract activity

Other sources of funding are available to providers, the significance of which varies according to local circumstances:

Extra contractual referrals

ECRs are patients seen for which a contract does not exist; they may be either emergency/urgent or elective admissions. The decision on which category is applicable in a particular case is left to clinical staff.

Providers bill the purchaser responsible for the treatment cost of an emergency/ urgent ECR and the purchaser is obliged to pay without questioning the need for admission or treatment. For non-emergency admissions, providers must seek prior authorization from the relevant purchaser. If such authorization is not obtained, then the purchaser is under no obligation to pay. Providers must publish each year a tariff of their ECR prices, specifically giving a charge for such items as a simple overnight stay for observation. Purchasers can use this list of tariffs to verify the charge made.

Service increment for teaching and research

SIFTR is provided to contribute to the costs of training and the carrying out of research. These costs are significant in providers with teaching responsibilities and have traditionally been funded as part of their operating costs. The introduction of contracts which link income to activity means that, to carry out its previous level of training and research, a provider would have to charge relatively higher prices than a competitor which does not undertake these activities. There is also the temptation for providers to cut their costs, and hence prices, by reducing their training and research activity. To avoid possible price distortions and prevent reductions in these activities these costs are removed from pricing descisions by funding them separately.

Financial planning and control

RHAs have the duty to create a framework for planning and to vet the plans of DHAs and FHSAs to ensure they are viable. These plans, together with that of the RHA itself, are then consolidated at the level of the RHA to provide an overall plan.

NHSTs prepare, on an annual basis, a rolling business plan covering the next three financial years. These should include details of the assumptions about inflation, workload, capital investment and risk. These plans are vetted by the NHSME.

Once plans have been agreed, they act as the control document against which the actual outturn can be judged. The comparison of the actual with the forecast results is also a valuable input to the next round of the planning cycle.

Conclusion

The NHS is an extremely large organization which must be subdivided if it is to be managed effectively. In doing this, a balance must be struck between giving central guidance and allowing local autonomy. This chapter has shown how this is achieved by explaining the overall structure of the NHS and the regulation of the relationship between the various parts. In particular, the process by which funds are introduced at the top and converted into direct patient care should be appreciated, together with how contracts are used to share the available funds between competing alternatives.

Questions

1. Outline the structure of the NHS and explain the means by which funds provided to the DoH are converted into patient care.
2. Why do capital charges not affect the aggregate amount of money spent by the NHS?
3. Identify and differentiate between the roles of purchasers and providers of health care in the NHS.
4. What types of contract can exist between purchasers and providers of health care?
   How certain can purchasers be of their total expenditure and providers of their total income once contracts for a year have been agreed?
5. What problems are created by the existence of activities which are not covered by contracts, and how are these problems overcome?

3

Cash flows and resource flows

AIMS

Accountancy is a system for recording and reporting transactions, in financial terms, so that interested parties can use this information as the basis for performance assessment and decision-making. Accountants apply rules, known as accounting concepts, when preparing accounting reports, and users must appreciate these if they are to be able to use the reports in a meaningful way. Accounting reports are built on the initial records of activity which give rise to transactions; similar transactions are then summarized, processed and reported. The general position is shown in Figure 3.1.

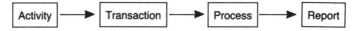

Figure 3.1 From activity to accounting report.

The operation of the flow shown in Figure 3.1 can be explained by means of an example. The employment of a nurse could be the activity, which is undertaken because the particular skills which the nurse can provide are needed to carry out the objectives of the organization, that is to deliver health care. At regular intervals, usually monthly, the nurse is paid, giving rise to a transaction which is recorded as part of the routine payroll operation. The processing through which this transaction is put enables a number of different reports to be prepared; some users require detailed information, while other are satisfied with more summarized data. At the most basic level, details of the pay of each individual employee must be kept. These can then be summarized in different ways to show the payroll costs of either different locations such as a ward, or different activities such as direct patient care.

This chapter deals with the measurement of resource flows and how this is linked to the related cash flows. The accounting reports prepared using the recorded details of resource and cash flows are dealt with elsewhere. After studying this chapter, readers will:

- be aware of the role of accounting concepts in the preparation of accounting reports;

- know the main accounting concepts;
- appreciate that, to carry out their function, organizations must have funds both to purchase long-term assets and finance day-to-day activities;
- understand how both long-term and short-term cash flows take place in an organization;
- recognize the links between resource flows and cash flows.

Measuring activity

It is clear to anyone looking at a hospital that it is a hive of activity. Patients arrive and depart, staff come on duty and go off duty, and supplies arrive, possibly go into the stores and are used. All of the activities can be looked on as flows, and the inflows and outflows which take place in a given period of time can be recorded and reported, together with any opening and closing stocks which exist at the start or end of the chosen period.

Table 3.1 shows a report on the set of flows related to waiting lists. Even though it is a very simple, non-financial, report, it contains elements common with the more complex accounting reports which will be considered later. It has an opening and closing position, and explains the changes which take place over the year in terms of inflows (new patients) and outflows (patients treated). Note how the balance between the inflows and outflows which take place during a period of time affects the closing position, and that the waiting list at the end of one year is the opening value for the next. Also, like accounting reports, its numerical accuracy and apparent simplicity can mask underlying complexity; those familiar with the compilation of waiting list statistics will be aware of how the information can be 'massaged', for example, one way of reporting a reduced number of inpatients waiting for treatment is to cut additions to the list by delaying the granting of initial outpatient appointments.

It can be seen how, in 19X8, the fact that more patients were treated than were added to the waiting list has caused the number of people waiting for treatment to decline over the year. The position is reversed in the following year when, although more patients were treated, the waiting list has grown because the number coming forward for treatment grew at a faster rate. Before any action could be taken in response to this report, further analysis would be needed to identify, at least, the behaviour of the waiting list for each specialty making up the total.

The size of the waiting list can also be expressed in terms of the amount of time

Table 3.1 Waiting lists and patient flows

	19X8	19X9
Opening patient stock	6 970	6 598
New patients	+83 437	+87 331
Total patient demand	90 407	93 929
Patients treated	−83 809	−86 744
Closing patient stock/waiting list	6 598	7 185

Table 3.2 A cash flow report

	19X1 £000	19X2 £000
Cash balance at start of year	24	36
Cash received	173 315	185 349
	173 339	185 385
Cash paid	−173 303	−185 402
Cash balance at end of year	36	−17

required to clear it, assuming future activity takes place at the same rate as in the past. For example, in Table 3.1 83 809 patients were treated in 19X8; this is an average of 6984 per month. Therefore, the waiting list of 6598 at the end of the year represents about one month's work.

We can now go on to look at a very simple accounting report and see how similar it is to the waiting list example. Table 3.2 shows a cash account which starts with the cash in hand and at bank at the start of a year, adds cash inflows and deducts cash outflows to leave the balance at the end of the year.

The report in Table 3.2 is useful in that it shows the overall movement, and the fact that a cash deficit has arisen at the end of the second year. However, it gives a very summarized picture, and analysis to show the sources of cash and the different ways in which it has been spent is needed before any decisions can be reached on how to deal with the deficit. A further deficiency is that it deals only with a single flow of resources and is open to manipulation. For example, to eliminate the cash deficit, it would be possible to delay paying a creditor for supplies until after the end of the second year. Although this would correct the reported overspend in cash terms, it means that a creditor exists at the year end, and is a first call on the cash available for the next year.

This example, based on cash flows, brings us to a very important distinction. Receipt or payment of a sum of cash is a fact which can be allocated to a particular accounting period, and it is important for the cash position to be monitored. In the NHS, it is not desirable, in the long run, to build up a large cash fund as this implies that it is not maximizing its possible activity, while cash deficits must also be avoided. Notwithstanding the use of cash as a focus, the accountant also aims to report the results of activity undertaken in an accounting period in an 'income and expenditure account', and the results shown in this are unlikely to coincide with the related cash flows. The accountant also prepares a 'balance sheet', which is a statement of an organization's assets and liabilities at a point in time.

Accounting operates in accordance with a set of concepts to select the flows and accumulations of value which are to be reported in financial terms and to determine the manner in which the report is compiled. These rules are not a set of immutable laws, but have developed over the years and been adapted as circumstances and requirements have changed. Anyone using financial reports must be aware that they are drawn up under these assumptions. In the private sector of the economy, State-ments of Standard Accounting Practice (SSAPs) and Financial Reporting Standards (FRSs) have been developed to specify how particular items must be dealt with for accounting purposes. The need for these regulations arose from the fact that different companies applied different rules when measuring similar items in their accounts, with the result that comparability between the accounts of companies was impaired. A number of SSAPs and FRSs have now been adopted by the NHS. Statement of Standard Accounting Practice 2 is applied in the NHS and lists four fundamental accounting concepts. These are:

Going concern concept

It is assumed that the entity is going to continue to exist into the foreseeable future. If it is not possible to assume this, then it implies that the entity is going to cease operating, and so assets have to be valued at what they could be sold for rather than at historical cost or replacement value. The application of this concept allows accountants to spread the value of an asset, by means of a depreciation charge, over the accounting periods expected to benefit from its use, rather than refer to its value on immediate disposal which, in the case of very specialized equipment, is likely to be limited to its value as scrap. Owing to the nature of its constitution, being established by statute, the going concern concept can be taken as applicable to the NHS.

Accruals concept

The financial impact of events is entered in the accounts as the events occur, and not when the related cash flow takes place. Some examples and consequences of this are:

- Goods received are recorded as purchases as they are received and not when they are paid for. Between the time of receipt and settlement they give rise to a creditor for the amount due, which is a liability.
- The value of fixed assets is spread over the accounting periods which benefit from their possession by means of a depreciation charge. The value of the asset not yet written off is carried in the balance sheet as an asset.
- Supplies, such as drugs, are charged against revenue when they are consumed, and **not** when they are purchased. Between the time of purchase and use they are recorded as an asset, stock.

The element common to the above examples is the recognition of the expenditure as a cost at the time of consumption, and not when the cash payment is made.

The accounts of some parts of the NHS depart from the accruals concept in respect of funding which is received in the form of the cash limit. This is, for the great part, provided by central government and the amount of cash which each procuring health authority is allowed to spend during a particular year is restricted by limiting the amount of cash which it can draw from the government's central account. For example, it is possible to obtain supplies on credit, and so include them as a charge in the current year (say 19X1) when they are consumed, but pay for them in the following year out of that year's (19X2) cash. The anticipated receipt of cash is not accrued in the year in which the supplies are charged (19X1), even though the benefit is received and consumed in that year.

Consistency concept

The same accounting treatment should be used to deal with similar items both within and between accounting periods. When preparing a set of accounts, all like items should be treated in the same way; for example, a consistent definition of what constitutes a fixed asset should be operated so that all such items are identified and included in the balance sheet. Once a particular approach has been adopted, it should then be applied in subsequent accounting periods. In the NHS, consistency is achieved because the form and content of the annual financial accounts are prescribed centrally.

Conservatism (or prudence) concept

This requires the accountant to make full provision for all expected costs as soon as it becomes apparent that they will arise, but not to anticipate income until it has been earned. For example, a fall in the value of items of stock to below cost should be recognized as it takes place, and not when the items are consumed. On the other hand, an increase in the value of items in stock due to an increase in their price is not shown in the accounts.

Other accounting concepts

There are a number of other concepts, in addition to those listed in SSAP 2 and explained above, which are applied when preparing accounting reports:

Entity concept

This fixes the boundary of the entity for which accounting reports are prepared. It is assumed that the accounting entity has an existence distinct from those employed in it, and the transactions are reported from the entity's point of view. In the NHS it is a requirement that the following entities maintain separate financial accounts:

- directly managed units
- district health authorities
- regional health authorities
- NHS trusts
- community health councils
- general practitioners
- family health service authorities.

It is possible to identify a number of other entities for which management accounting reports may be prepared – for example, reports may relate to an individual department or ward within a hospital. The form and content of these reports is subject to local discretion and it is important to know, both when preparing and using them, the entity and the time period to which they relate.

Money measurement concept

Items are included in the accounts only if a monetary value can be assigned to them with a reasonable degree of accuracy. A possible result of applying this concept is that some factors which have a significant impact on an entity's ability to fulfil its purpose may not be reflected in the accounts. For example, the possession of a team of specialists with an international reputation and the possession of a sophisticated information system are valuable assets for a hospital, but no value is assigned to them and they do not appear as assets in the hospital's accounting reports. On the other hand, a hospital's site is valued and reported in the balance sheet even though the ability of the hospital to deliver health care is more dependent on its personnel than, within certain limits, its location.

Realization concept

This is used to determine the amount of income an entity can take credit for in an accounting period. Income is usually realized when the organization has completed its side of the transaction, for example by providing the services agreed under a contract or carrying out an ECR. The entry of income in the accounts should not be anticipated, that is taken as earned before the event giving rise to the income has taken place. For example, a hospital may have a block contract producing agreed income of £50 000 per month for a year. It is not correct to include the whole of the year's income, £50 000 × 12 = £600 000, in the first month's accounts since the activity to earn the income for the subsequent eleven months has not yet taken place. As a result, accounts prepared for each of the twelve months covered by the contract would include one month's income, that is £50 000.

Matching concept

The outcome for a period of time, either a surplus or a deficit, is measured by matching the income generated during the period with the costs incurred to generate it. The first step is to identify the income, and the second step is to deduct from it the expenditures related to producing it. This concept shows how a number of the concepts are interrelated, as it is put into effect by applying the realization concept described above.

Materiality concept

Accounting statements should contain only those financial facts which are material, or relevant, to the decisions to be made by the user of the report. The consequences of this are:

- Accounts must be suited to the decisions to be taken by their users and their content can be tailored to meet the users' needs. For example, a trust chief executive is likely to be interested in the overall performance of the trust, analysed across the main management divisions. At a lower level of management, a clinical director would want a greater level of detail, for example the cost of each employee group for which he or she is responsible.

- Excessive detail should be avoided, and time saved, by not reporting trivia. For example, minor items of expenditure should be grouped together under a 'Sundry' or 'Miscellaneous' heading. Only if this figure is unexpectedly high should further analysis be undertaken.
- Summarization should not be taken too far. For example, the balance sheet should not contain a single heading 'Fixed assets' but should disclose separately the values of different types of assets, such as land, buildings and equipment.

The use of computerization means that it is possible for the accountant to produce summarized figures, and then, on request, provide further details of the items which comprise them. For example, the amount owed to a hospital for work carried out but not yet paid for is reported as a single figure 'Debtors'; interested managers could be provided with further analysis summarized by age of debt, or, if necessary, a complete list of all the separate amounts due could be produced.

Valuation

A decision has to be reached on how the transactions and assets of an entity are to be valued. The NHS uses two bases:

- **Historical cost.** This is applied to all items which are described as 'revenue' transactions. That is, they relate to the day-to-day running of the organization and include such costs as salaries and consumables such as drugs. These transactions are recorded at the amount of cash which is paid for them – that is, what they cost. It is also used to value assets, other than fixed assets, in the balance sheet, with the result that stocks are valued at their cost, even if they have gone up in price between the date of purchase and the balance sheet date. A great advantage of using historical cost is that it is based on fact; it is possible to refer to the invoice or other payment record to find the amount paid for an item and hence verify its value for accounting purposes. The obvious deficiency is that, in a time of changing prices, the historical cost becomes an out-of-date measure of the asset's worth.
- **Current value.** The longer the period of time between the acquisition of an asset and the date on which a balance sheet is being prepared, the greater the divergence is likely to be between its original cost and its current worth. This difference is likely to be especially marked in the case of fixed assets, which are those with a high cost and an expectation to give benefit to a number of accounting periods. In the NHS, they are recorded at cost when they are bought, but are subsequently revalued to their current replacement cost when a balance sheet is prepared.

It is from a failure to appreciate the existence and application of these accounting concepts that a lot of the misconceptions surrounding accounting reports arise. The terminology of accounting uses words in common everyday usage, but gives them specialized meanings. For example, at first consideration, the 'receipts and payments account' may appear to convey the same information as an 'income and expenditure account', but the former contains only cash flows while the latter applies the accruals and other accounting concepts to report the values attached to the activities which have taken place in the specified time period. This emphasizes the need to know **what is being measured** in accounting reports and **how it has been valued.** Bearing this in mind, we can now go on to consider the cash flows of an organization.

The role of cash

It is essential for any organization to be able to settle its debts as they fall due. In the short term this means having money available to pay for wages and salaries, heating and lighting, consumable stores, and all the other ongoing running costs. The longer term also has to be considered, as capital assets have to be paid for and loans repaid. If an organization runs out of cash, it is possible to make use of an overdraft, but this is purely a short-term measure. In the NHS, the government requires that providers keep their costs within their income, and would not allow an ever-increasing overdraft to be used. Therefore, where it appears that a cash deficit is likely to arise, action is taken either to reduce outflows or increase inflows so as to bring the position back into balance.

We can now look in more detail at the cash flows which take place within an NHS health care provider. This is shown in Figure 3.2, which relates to a simplified model of an NHS trust hospital. Note how the flows, although all centred on cash, are divided between long term and short term; these are now each considered in more detail.

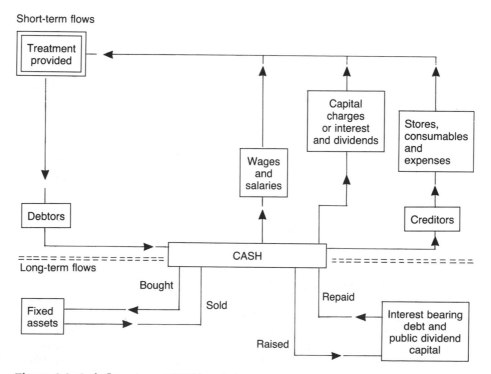

Figure 3.2 Cash flows in an NHST hospital.

Long-term flows

The prime objective of a hospital is to provide treatment to patients, and, to do this, it has to spend money. First of all facilities are needed, such as land, buildings, and plant and equipment; once these have been acquired, staff and other costs must be paid so that the facilities can function. As a general rule, assets which are expected to last for a long time should be purchased from funds which either do not have to be repaid, such as public dividend capital, or are not due for repayment until some considerable time in the future, such as interest bearing debt. The routine running costs can be met out of current income as it is generated.

Central government maintains a division between funds which it supplies for the purchase of capital assets and those which are for running the service, although a limited amount of transfer between them, known as virement, is allowed. When a directly managed hospital wants to buy additional fixed assets, it must make a bid for some of the available capital funds, and, if it is successful, the money will be allocated to it. NHS trusts obtain funds for capital spending from internally generated sources or permitted borrowing. In the NHS the vast bulk of investment in long-term assets already exists, and was financed over the years by capital funds from the government. Another way to obtain capital funds is to sell an existing fixed asset, and this can raise significant amounts where property is concerned. The proportion of the proceeds which the selling unit is allowed to keep depends on the particular arrangements, but significant disposals are often part of large overall development schemes, in which circumstances the money raised would be reinvested locally.

Capital spending shows up in the balance sheet as an increase in the total described as 'Fixed assets', but more detailed information is required by management to monitor the day-to-day progress of its capital programme. The accounting reports needed for this purpose show the total amount allocated for the purchase less the total of cash spent to date plus anticipated future expenditure to completion. This balance demonstrates whether the asset will be acquired within the allocated budget.

These reports are straightforward in the case of a single fixed asset, such as a piece of equipment, but greater complexity occurs where the acquisition takes place over a number of years, as happens when a new hospital is built. Comparison of the reports over the years is likely to reveal variations, which is to be expected because long-term cash flows tend to be 'lumpy', that is one year might see a high value of capital transactions while in the next there are hardly any.

The amount of analysis contained in the reports depends on the purpose for which they are required. Detailed accounts are needed for each individual asset to monitor the progress of its acquisition. At the other extreme, summaries are sufficient to demonstrate to higher management that the capital programme is on course.

Short-term flows

The flows in Figure 3.2 show the cash effects of treating patients. Supplies are purchased, with an immediate outflow if they are for cash, or a later outflow if a period of credit is taken. DMUs have to pay capital charges, which comprise interest on the value of their fixed assets plus a depreciation charge to reflect their loss in value over the accounting period. Trusts pay interest and dividends on their long-term funds used to finance their fixed assets, but their depreciation charges are not matched by a cash outflow; this feature of depreciation charges is returned to later. Staff payments can be assumed to be contemporaneous with the hospital deriving the benefit from employment in the form of services. All of these outflows have the final aim of providing treatment for patients.

The bulk of cash inflows is generated by providing treatment under contracts with health care purchasers. The cash consequences of the different types of contract are:

- **Block contracts.** The hospital receives an annual sum, in instalments, and in exchange gives access to a defined range of services. The contract should include agreement on the cash payments to be made and their timing, and so the provider has a predetermined amount of cash receivable throughout the period.
- **Cost and volume contracts.** A baseline level of activity, measured in treatments or cases, is provided in exchange for a set sum. Subject to a tolerance level, commonly agreed at between 2% and 5%, if the number of cases treated in more or less than the agreed number, the total payment is varied to reflect this. This type of contract therefore generates a set minimum cash inflow, with the possibility of marginal adjustments subject to the volume of cases treated.
- **Cost per case.** This is for use in circumstances not covered by the other two types of contract. Payment is made on a case-by-case basis, and is not subject to any commitment, by either party, about the volume of such work. The cash flow from this type of contract, and that from ECRs, is therefore irregular and cannot be forecast with any degree of accuracy.

Cash may also be received from:

- charitable donations
- the treatment of private patients
- the provision of services, such as pathology, to other units
- sales in the staff dining-room
- secondary income, for example car park charges
- interest on invested cash balances.

The relationship between cash flows and resource flows

Accounting reports which deal with flows of resources into and out of the organization have to relate to a period of time. The income and expenditure account contains the resource flows, and the cash account the cash flows. In many cases the cash flow and the associated economic event both take place during the same accounting period; for example, a hospital, whether a DMU or a trust, draws up its annual accounts to 31 March and so, for example, both the flow of cash outwards in January for the payment of wages and the flow of benefit derived from them are completed in the same period. In other cases, the economic event and its cash flows arise in different accounting periods, and so it is not sufficient to report only the cash flows, as this ignores the accounting concept of accruals whereby reports are based on the economic events which have taken place during a period. This is illustrated in Figure 3.3.

Figure 3.3 represents the accounting year to 31 March 19X2 along the central line. Both the cost of the supplies and the income from the treatment of the ECR patient

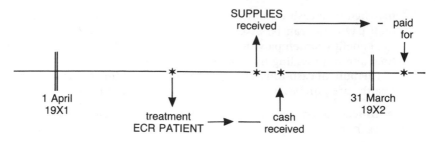

Figure 3.3 Reporting resource flows and cash flows.

are reflected in the income and expenditure account for the year to 31 March 19X2, but only the cash received for treating the patient appears in that year's cash account. The cash payment for the supplies is recorded and reported in the cash account for the year to 31 March 19X3. Management must use both the income and expenditure account and cash account as measures of activity as the income and expenditure account must remain broadly in balance, and, at the same time, unfunded cash deficits must be avoided.

It is important to appreciate the fact that an economic event and its cash flow may be reported in different accounting periods and that it is not sufficient to monitor only one of these aspects, as the behaviour of one is not necessarily reflected in that of the other. In some cases, concentrating on one of them to the detriment of the other can result in serious consequences. For example, the acquisition of fixed assets by an NHS trust is not immediately reflected in the income and expenditure account but is an immediate drain on cash resources. In these circumstances, failure to monitor the cash account is likely to mean that cash runs out and, at best, expensive emergency funds have to be borrowed; at worst, bills remain unpaid, supplies are cut off, and suppliers take legal action.

We can now go on to consider the usual cases where resource flows and cash flows take place in different accounting periods, and the manner in which the two flows are linked.

Debtors

Debtors arise when income is generated, for example by treating a patient, but the cash is not received immediately. A debtor exists between the time the payment becomes due and the receipt of cash. The result is that the income for a given period of time is not equal to the cash received; these two measures are linked by the opening and closing debtors, as shown in Figure 3.4.

Figure 3.4 shows an accounting year which runs up to 31 March 19X2 and the income and cash received related to three treatments. In the case of treatment 1, the income arises prior to 1 April 19X1 and the cash is received afterwards so that a debtor exists at the start of the accounting period; this means that some of the cash received in the year to 31 March 19X2 relates to income shown in the income and expenditure account of the previous year. Both cash and income from treatment 2 are recorded in the same year. The income from treatment 3 is included as income in

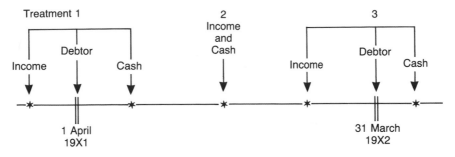

Figure 3.4 The link between income and cash received.

the current year, but the cash due is not settled until the following one. In summary, the cash and income statements for the year to 31 March 19X2 will report:

● Cash: Treatments 1 and 2 (1 being an opening debtor);
● Income: Treatments 2 and 3 (3 being a closing debtor).

This shows that the difference between cash received and income is caused by the existence of both opening and closing debtors, and it is possible, given the values of opening and closing debtors and either income or cash received, to calculate the missing figure. The relationship can be expressed generally as:

	Formula	Numerical example £000		Formula	Numerical example £000
	Cash received	5600		Income	5690
−	Opening debtors	(350)	+	Opening debtors	350
+	Closing debtors	440	−	Closing debtors	(440)
=	Income	5690	=	Cash received	5600

Creditors

Creditors are created when there is a time lag between the receipt of goods or services purchased from outside the unit and when the cash is paid to settle the debt. It is not necessary to draw a diagram again, as by referring to Figure 3.4 it is possible to imagine the receipt of three lots of supplies:

● Lot 1 is received prior to 31 March 19X1 and is paid for after that date; this gives rise to an opening creditor.
● Lot 2 is received and paid for during the current year.
● Lot 3 is received during the current year and paid for in the next one, so that there is a closing creditor at 31 March 19X2.

Each lot is reflected in the cash and purchases reports for the year to 31 March 19X2 as follows:

- Cash:　　Lots 1 and 2 (1 being an opening creditor);
- Purchases: Lots 2 and 3 (3 being a closing creditor).

The cash and purchases reports coincide only in respect of those items purchased and paid for during the accounting period. In general, the link between the two flows is given by the formula:

	Formula	Numerical example £000		Formula	Numerical example £000
	Cash paid	1360		Purchases	1450
−	Opening creditors	(500)	+	Opening creditors	500
+	Closing creditors	590	−	Closing creditors	(590)
=	Purchases	1450	=	Cash paid	1360

Stocks

The value of purchases made during a year does not reflect fully the amount of an item actually consumed; to find this, and hence the entry in the income and expenditure account, it is necessary to adjust for opening and closing stocks. To see the impact of this, consider the stocks of drugs kept in a pharmacy, as shown in Figure 3.5.

At the start of the accounting year there exists a stock of drugs which is counted and valued; this stock is part of the consumption in the year to 31 March 19X2. Throughout the accounting year, further purchases are made; some of these, in the above example 80%, are used up, while others, the balance of 20%, are held in stock at the year end. Therefore, to find the amount consumed during the year, the opening stock has to be added to purchases, and the closing stock deducted. The general formula is:

	Formula	Numerical example £000		Formula	Numerical example £000
	Purchases	875		Cost of items consumed	850
+	Opening stocks	120	−	Opening stocks	(120)
−	Closing stocks	(145)	+	Closing stocks	145
=	Cost of items consumed	850	=	Purchases	875

Prepayments

Prepayments occur where a payment is made to receive a service for a period of time which overlaps the accounting date. For example, rent of £10 000 may be paid for

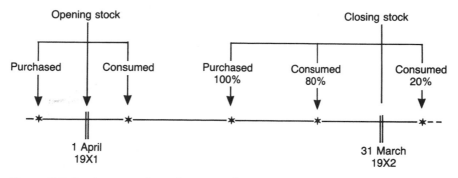

Figure 3.5 Purchases, stocks and consumption.

six months in advance on 1 January 19X2. This gives the right to occupy premises up to 30 June 19X2, and so, at the accounting date of 31 March, half of the benefit, worth £5000, has still to be received. Looked at another way, the income and expenditure account should only show the rent for the year to 31 March. Where there is a closing prepayment, there is likely also to be an opening one, and very often these cancel each other out. The expenditure related to a service, for which payment is made in advance, to be shown in the income and expenditure account, is linked to the cash paid for the period as follows:

	Formula	Numerical example £		Formula	Numerical example £
	Cash paid	4200		Expenditure	4000
+	Opening prepayment	500	−	Opening prepayment	(500)
−	Closing prepayment	(700)	+	Closing prepayment	700
=	Expenditure	4000	=	Cash paid	4200

The opening prepayment was paid in cash in the previous year, but gives benefits to the current one, while the closing prepayment is caused by a cash outflow in the current period which gives benefits to the next one.

Accruals

Accruals are similar to prepayments, but arise when items are paid for in arrears. For example, electricity is billed after it has been used, and it is likely that consumption for March will not be billed and paid for until after the end of the month. To determine the cost of consumption for a given period of time, amounts used but not paid for must be included. However, the first amount paid at the start of the period is likely to be for usage during the last part of the previous period. The link between usage and cash flow for a given period is:

	Formula	Numerical example £		Formula	Numerical example £
	Cash paid	9000		Consumption	9800
−	Opening accrual	(1200)	+	Opening accrual	1200
+	Closing accrual	2000	−	Closing accrual	(2000)
=	Consumption	9800	=	Cash paid	9000

Assume that the above example relates to electricity consumption, the accounting year runs to 31 March 19X2, and electricity is billed three monthly in arrears. The opening accrual relates to usage for the first three months of 19X1, which was paid for in April of that year; as the economic benefit was received in the financial year to 31 March 19X1, its cost is charged in its income and expenditure account, while its cash effect arises in the subsequent year. The consumption in January, February and March 19X2 has to be included in the income and expenditure account of the year to the end of March, although it is not paid until the next year.

Depreciation

Although the final item considered in this section, depreciation is one which causes a major difference between the cash flows of a period and reported expenditure. A fixed asset is one which has a long life and is acquired with the objective of retaining it within the organization. Fixed assets are needed to provide the infrastructure, and they are used up over their lifetime. The matching and accruals concepts require that the cost of using resources is included in the income and expenditure account when the economic benefit is received, and not when the related cash payment takes place. Therefore, the cost of fixed assets is charged, not when they are acquired, but over their lives. Each year that benefits from the ownership of a fixed asset bears a related cost in the form of a depreciation charge. This is illustrated in Figure 3.6.

Figure 3.6 shows the acquisition of an asset in the year to 31 March 19X1, which gives equal benefits to the year of purchase and the next four, that is it has an expected life of five years. The financial effect of the acquisition in the form of a cash

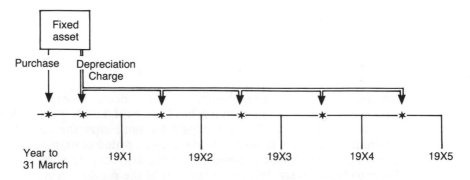

Figure 3.6 Fixed assets and the depreciation charge.

outflow takes place in the first year, but its consumption is reflected in the income and expenditure accounts of each of the five years for which it is in service by means of a depreciation charge. The valuation of fixed assets and the calculation of the depreciation charge are considered later.

Fixed assets

Fixed assets are also known as 'capital assets', and are defined as those which are tangible and capable of being used for a period exceeding one year. However, the strict application of this definition would lead to the inclusion of minor items, such as pencil sharpeners, and it is obviously not cost effective to subject the trivial amounts involved in such purchases to the full process of accounting for fixed assets. This problem is overcome by applying the concept of materiality. In order to achieve uniformity throughout the NHS, the level at which an acquisition is deemed material is set in cash terms, and fixed assets are currently defined as those with a life in excess of one year and cost in excess of £5000. This value is likely to be increased over time in response to rises in the cost of assets. Items which are within the theoretical definition of fixed assets, but cost less than the financial limit, are written off to the income and expenditure account, either at the time of purchase, or of consumption if classified as stock items.

Once a fixed asset is acquired, it is likely that further expenditure will have to be made to keep it in good repair. These costs are written off to the income and expenditure account as they are incurred. There is a grey area between what is maintenance and what is expenditure on improving fixed assets, especially if upgrading takes place at the same time as a programme of maintenance. This can cause problems as the expenditure on upgrading should be added to the value of the fixed asset. There is no simple solution to this difficulty, and each case must be judged on its individual facts.

Control over fixed assets is maintained by the use of a capital asset register. This is a record in which each fixed asset is identified separately together with such information as its:

- location
- date of acquisition
- initial cost
- expected life and likely date of replacement
- maintenance requirements.

To keep the register up to date, systems must be established to ensure that all new assets are entered in it at the time they are acquired, and the entries relating to all disposals are removed. As part of the audit function, checks can be made that assets listed in the register are still possessed, and that all acquisitions and disposals have been properly authorized.

After all the fixed assets have been identified and entered in the register, the accounting questions of how to value them and calculate an annual charge for their use have to be addressed. In general terms, the basis of valuation used is current replacement cost, and the use of fixed assets gives rise to a depreciation charge. The application of this approach to a particular asset depends on its type, and, in the NHS, fixed assets are divided into four categories:

- **Land** is valued by the district valuer every three years. In between valuations, revaluation is approximated every quarter by applying an appropriate index. No depreciation is charged in respect of freehold land because it is not 'used up' or worn out as a result of being used to deliver health care.
- **Buildings,** including fixed services such as lifts, are revalued every three years with intervening quarterly indexation. The expected life will be set at the time of the triennial revaluation, and will not exceed 80 years. However, if the building is well maintained and showing no signs of deterioration, its life expectancy can be uprated at the time of each revaluation. This is important because a longer life results in a lower annual depreciation charge since there is a longer period of time over which to recover the value of the asset.
- **Equipment** is divided into broad categories, each of which is revalued to current replacement cost every quarter using an index appropriate to the type of asset. Standard lives of each type of asset are provided, and these are used to calculate the depreciation charge.
- **Assets under construction** are projects which will result in the possession of a fixed asset when they are completed. Currently, they are valued at expenditure to date plus compound interest, calculated on a quarterly basis using the value at the start of the quarter, and are not depreciated. The calculation of the value of an asset under construction is shown in Figure 3.7. This approach is subject to review.

In all cases, where it is intended to dispose of a fixed asset, the valuation should be based on how much it is expected to raise.

The depreciation charge is calculated using straight line depreciation. This is found by dividing the current value of the asset, however determined, by its anticipated

An asset costs in total £4 million and is to be built over the course of a year with a payment of £1 million being made each quarter. The annual rate of interest is 6%. The value of the asset is calculated as follows:

Quarter	1 £m	2 £m	3 £m	4 £m
Value at start of quarter	–	1.000	2.015	3.045
Additional expenditure in quarter	1.000	1.000	1.000	1.000
	1.000	2.000	3.015	4.045
Interest	–	0.015	0.030	0.046
Value at end of quarter	1.000	2.015	3.045	4.091

Notes:
1. The annual rate of interest is 6%, and so the rate applicable to each quarter is 1.5%.
2. The amount of interest added each quarter is calculated on the value at the start of the quarter.
3. The completed asset, valued at £4.091 million, is transferred to the appropriate balance sheet heading, and depreciated from the time it is brought into use.

Figure 3.7 Valuation of an asset under construction.

An asset is bought for £10 000 on 1 April 19X1. It is expected to have a life of ten years, and be worth nothing at the end.

The increase in its replacement cost is zero for the first five years of its life, but in the sixth year it increases by 10%.

Its capital charges for the fifth and sixth years of its life, the years to 31 March 19X6 and 19X7, are:

Year to 31 March	19X6 £	19X7 £	Note
Replacement cost at start of year	10 000	10 000	
Revaluation during year	0	1 000	1
Replacement cost at end of year	10 000	11 000	
Accumulated depreciation at start of year	4 000	5 000	
Revaluation	0	500	1
Charge for year	1 000	1 100	2,5
Accumulated depreciation at end of year	5 000	6 600	
Written down value at end of year	5 000	4 400	3
Interest at 6% on year-end value	300	264	4,5

Notes:
1. Both the cost and accumulated depreciation brought forward are increased by 10%.
2. The charge for the year is 10% of the asset's replacement cost. Both NHSTs and non-trusts charge this in the income and expenditure account.
3. The written-down value appears in the balance sheet and is the replacement cost, less accumulated depreciation.
4. Non-trusts calculate notional interest on the written-down value of capital assets owned and charge it in the income and expenditure account.
5. Non-trusts pay a sum equal to their capital charges to their RHA.

Figure 3.8 Calculation of capital charges.

life, and the resulting cost is entered in the income and expenditure account. In the balance sheet, fixed assets are shown at their revalued amount, less accumulated depreciation, which is the total of all the annual depreciation charges which have previously been made in respect of the asset. The calculation of capital charges is illustrated in Figure 3.8.

In practice, the revaluation – and for non-trusts interest – calculations are performed on a quarterly basis, with the result that the calculations are more complex than those shown in Figure 3.8. Depreciation and interest charges included in accounting reports are based on these more complex calculations, and an example of their operation is given by question 1 at the end of this chapter.

It is likely that the life of an asset will not in fact be the same as that assumed for calculating the depreciation charge. For example, a fixed asset may be written off over ten years for depreciation purposes, but actually last 12 years. However, by writing off 10% of its value each year, the total depreciation charged at the end of its tenth year will be equal to its value, and so it will have a written-down value of zero; these are known as 'fully depreciated' assets. Its value and accumulated depreciation should be maintained in the balance sheet for the eleventh and twelfth years of its life while it is still in use, and then, when it is taken out of service, both of these balances should be removed.

If, when an asset is disposed of, any proceeds are received, then these should be compared with its written-down value and the surplus or deficit on disposal calculated. A deficit on disposal indicates that not enough depreciation has been charged in previous years, while a surplus shows the opposite. The fact that too much or too little depreciation has been charged over the years means that the entries in the income and expenditure account have been wrong; this inaccuracy has

	£000	Note
Gross replacement cost at 1 April 19X1	52 000	1
Additions	1 360	
Indexation	420	2
Disposals	(190)	
Gross replacement cost at 31 March 19X2	53 590	
Accumulated depreciation at 1 April 19X1	10 390	1
Charge for the year	1 086	3
Indexation	92	2
Disposals	(150)	4
Accumulated depreciation at 31 March 19X2	11 418	
Net book value at 31 March 19X2	42 172	5

Notes:
1. These values are found from the closing balance sheet of the previous year, that is the balance sheet for 31 March 19X1.
2. The indexation changes the opening values in line with increases in value which have taken place during the whole year, and from the date of acquisition to the year end for assets bought during the year. The accumulated depreciation has to be indexed so that it is consistent with the replacement cost on which the annual charge is based.
3. This is the same value as that entered as the charge for depreciation in the income and expenditure account and represents the value of fixed assets consumed during the current year.
4. The depreciation related to assets disposed of has to be removed from the accounts as well as its current replacement cost; once an asset is no longer owned, all the accounting entries relating to it must be eliminated.
5. This is the value included in the balance sheet.

Figure 3.9 Opening and closing values of fixed assets.

to be accepted as inherent in a system of accounting based on estimates of asset lives and valuations. The position is corrected, to some extent, by entering the surplus or deficit on disposal, when it is identified, in the income and expenditure account.

The fact that fixed assets last for more than one year means that an individual asset will constitute part of the total value of fixed assets in a number of consecutive balance sheets. However, the value at which it is included will not be the same because each year it is both revalued and depreciated. To explain the linkage between the opening and closing values of fixed assets, a note has to be attached to the balance sheet showing all of the separate movements which have caused the overall change. An outline of this note, including indicative values, is given in Figure 3.9.

Conclusion

This chapter has identified flows of resources, related them to their cash impact and showed how both the cash effect and economic effect are calculated. It also looked at the processes used to measure activity prior to its inclusion in accounting reports, and showed the valuation techniques to be applied. The following chapter reviews the main accounting reports and demonstrates how they are used to report the activity and position of the entity to which they relate.

Questions

*1. The following information relates to a capital asset which was purchased in quarter 1 and brought into use during quarter 2:

(i)   Cost £1 000 000;
(ii) Expected life of five years (20 quarters);
(iii) Index numbers for the first four quarters are:

Quarter	[1]	[2]	[3]	[4]
Opening index number	100	101	103	103
Closing index number	101	103	103	110

(iv) Annual interest charge 6%.

Required:

(a) Assuming the asset was purchased by an NHST, calculate the depreciation charge for its first year of use and its value to be included in the balance sheet at the end of the year.
(b) Explain the consequences if the asset was purchased by a non-NHST.

2. What do you understand by the term 'accounting concepts', and what is their role in the accounting process?

Explain and illustrate the application of the following accounting concepts to the NHS:

- going concern
- accruals

- consistency
- conservatism
- entity
- money measurement
- realization
- matching
- materiality.

*3. Define the term 'debtors'.

   Explain why an organization's cash received and income for a period of time are not necessarily equal in value.

   At the start of the year, an NHST has debtors of £800 000, during the year it fulfils contracts to the value of £9 600 000, and at the end of the year debtors are £950 000. How much cash did the trust receive during the year in respect of contracts?

4. What is a 'depreciation charge', and why is it included in the income and expenditure account?

5. Differentiate between long-term and short-term flows of cash, and explain why this distinction is important.

4

Accounting statements

AIMS

The previous chapter examined the links between resource flows and cash flows. On an annual basis, these flows have to be summarized and reported in accordance with the requirements of the DoH. These reports relate to the entity as a whole, and their production is part of the financial accounting process which shows how the resources provided to the separate parts of the NHS have been used. The information contained in the annual reports is publicly available, and does not go into very great detail. This is in contrast to the management accounts which are only for internal use and are designed to enable managers to control the activities for which they are responsible. As a result, management accounting reports contain a great amount of detail, but deal with only the part of the organization for which the manager is responsible. It is logical that the overall picture presented in the financial accounts is the sum of the detailed management accounts relating to all the constituent parts of the entity, and, to avoid unnecessary duplication, it is preferable to operate an integrated system of management and financial accounts.

This chapter deals with the production of financial accounting statements which relate to individual entities within the NHS such as an NHST hospital. Similar statements can be prepared for parts within entities, such as a catering department, or they can be consolidated to show the results for larger sections. Whatever part or subdivision of the NHS they relate to, accounting reports present a financial picture, and, to derive benefit from them, users must be able to interpret them; this relies on understanding how they are constructed. The aims of this chapter are to:

- introduce the main accounting statements: balance sheet, income and expenditure account and cash flow statement;
- show how to prepare the main accounting statements;
- explain the links between the main accounting statements;
- develop a worked example, including the receipts and payment account.

It is a requirement that the annual accounts of an entity for its second and subsequent years of operation include 'comparative figures' for the previous year. This means that an extra column is included in the accounts which contains the corresponding values taken from the accounts of the previous year. This provides a basis for comparing the results of the current year and judging the organization's relative progress. Although the provision of the figures for two consecutive years is useful, it is too short a period of time to determine whether particular trends have been established, and, to do this, the accounts for a number of years should be used. In this chapter, comparative figures have been omitted from all the examples.

The balance sheet

The balance sheet is an accounting statement which contains the values of the assets and liabilities of an entity at a point in time. In the NHS, it shows the aggregate written-down replacement cost of the fixed assets plus the value of working capital. The total value it reveals must not be mistaken for the value which the entity could be sold for as a whole, since this depends on what a buyer is willing to pay for it, and this, in turn, is usually related to the amount which can be generated from owning and running the entity.

The balance sheet also explains how the entity has funded the assets which it owns. Figure 4.1 contains two simplified balance sheets, one for a DMU and the other for an NHS trust, showing how fixed assets are financed. It is clear that the value of assets is equal to the value of liabilities, which, in this instance, is represented by the funds provided in the form of capital and debt. The fact that assets are equal in value to liabilities is a fundamental balance sheet rule and is the natural consequence of operating a system of double-entry book-keeping. This rule will hold no matter what transactions are undertaken, and failure for a balance sheet to balance in this way indicates that an error has been made.

In the case of the DMU in Figure 4.1, the Capital account represents the funds invested by the health authority which manages it. In the case of the trust, the balance on the Capital account has been converted to amounts due to the Department of Health, and comprises a mixture of the following:

- **Public dividend capital (PDC)** is a form of long-term finance, that is it does not have to be repaid. It does not carry an obligation for repayment or interest charges, but, in the long run, dividend payments, which are a form of interest, are expected at a rate at least equal to that on Interest bearing debt.
- **Interest bearing debt (IBD)** carries a fixed interest charge and is subject to repayment in the longer term.

The ratio between these two types of finance is negotiated individually for each

	DMU £000	Trust £000
Fixed assets		
Land and buildings	20 000	20 000
Equipment	4 000	4 000
	24 000	24 000
Financed by:		
Capital account	24 000	
Public dividend capital		12 000
Interest bearing debt		12 000
	24 000	24 000

Figure 4.1 Financing fixed assets.

	DMU £000	Trust £000
Fixed assets		
Land and buildings	21 000	21 000
Equipment	4 500	4 500
	25 500	25 500
Financed by:		
Capital account	25 500	
Public dividend capital		12 000
Interest bearing debt		12 000
Revaluation reserve		1 500
	25 500	25 500

Figure 4.2 The effects of revaluation.

NHST, and the rates of dividend on PDC and interest on IBD are set so as to give an overall return of 6%.

Another way of looking at the section of the balance sheet which shows how the assets have been financed is that it represents the amount due to 'ownership'; it is the amount which ownership has invested in the entity. As a result, any changes in the values of assets is reflected in this value. For example, Figure 4.2 shows what happens if the assets in Figure 4.1 are revalued to £21 million for land and buildings and £4.5 million for equipment. In the DMU, the increase in value is added to the Capital account, while the trust has to open a new account in which to record the effects of revaluations.

To achieve long-term financial stability, fixed assets, which are going to be held for a considerable period of time, should be funded by long-term sources of finance. Failure to do this will result in liquidity problems. For example, the trust shown in Figure 4.2 owns a significant quantity of assets, but, since it has no cash, it is not in a position to make any payments. The use of short-term funds to buy fixed assets would have meant that it could not make the repayments when due without selling off some of the fixed assets.

NHS trusts are created by taking over existing assets and liabilities, and so the initial balance sheet will look more like that in Figure 4.3 although currently they do not inherit cash.

An obvious point looking at the balance sheet in Figure 4.3 is that the value of net assets, £24 140 000, is equal to the total sources of finance. This is another example of the rule that assets must be equal in value to liabilities. It also shows that the acquisition of assets requires a source of funds. This fact is illustrated in Figure 4.4 which reports the effect on the balance sheet from Figure 4.3 of raising additional IBD of £1 000 000 to buy new equipment. The values of both Total assets less current liabilities and Total finance increase by £1 000 000 to £25 140 000.

It is now possible to consider the impact on the balance sheet of undertaking activity. Starting from the position in Figure 4.4, assume that in the month of April 19X2 income of £2 400 000 was earned and all received in cash, and expenses, such

	£000	£000
Fixed assets		
Land and buildings		20 000
Plant and equipment		4 000
		24 000
Current assets		
Stocks	200	
Debtors	120	
Cash in hand and at bank	50	
	370	
Current liabilities		
Creditors	230	
Net current assets		140
Total assets less current liabilities		24 140
Financed by:		
Public dividend capital		12 070
Interest bearing debt		12 070
Total finance		24 140

Figure 4.3 NHS trust balance sheet at 1 April 19X2.

as wages and drugs, of £2 300 000 were paid in cash. For simplicity, also assume that no changes took place in the values of stock, debtors or creditors; these will be dealt with later. The depreciation charge for the month is £26 000 for buildings and £41 000 for equipment. The surplus for the month is:

	£000	£000
Income		2400
Expenses	2300	
Depreciation	67	
		2367
Surplus		33

The cash balance at the end of the month is:

	£000
Balance at 1 April	50
Receipts	2400
Payments	−2300
Balance at 30 April	150

	£000	£000
Fixed assets		
Land and buildings		20 000
Plant and equipment		5 000
		25 000
Current assets		
Stocks	200	
Debtors	120	
Cash in hand and at bank	50	
	370	
Current liabilities		
Creditors	230	
Net current assets		140
Total assets less current liabilities		25 140
Financed by:		
Public dividend capital		12 070
Interest bearing debt		13 070
Total finance		25 140

Figure 4.4 NHS trust balance sheet at 1 April 19X2.

Note that the cash balance has increased by £100 000, while the surplus in the income and expenditure account is only £33 000. The difference is explained by the fact that, for an NHS trust, the depreciation charge is a non-cash expense, that is it does not result in a cash outflow. The cash retained is at the disposal of management, and can be used for current or future developments which require additional, or replacement, assets to be acquired.

The balance sheet for the end of the month can now be drawn up, and appears in Figure 4.5.

The income and expenditure account

A new heading appears in the balance sheet in Figure 4.5 compared with Figure 4.4, namely 'Income and expenditure account'. During the month of April 19X2, a surplus of £33 000 was made, and, as this is a long-term source of finance, it is added to the initial investment of public dividend capital and long-term loans. Subsequent surpluses will be added to this account, and deficits deducted from it. The income and expenditure account contains details of the resources earned and used up during an accounting period. Figure 4.6 shows a typical income and expenditure account for either a DMU or an NHS trust.

The format and contents of the accounts and financial returns to be submitted are specified by the Department of Health. Figure 4.6 is sufficient to show the principle

	£000	£000
Land and buildings:		
at replacement cost	20 000	
less accumulated depreciation	26	19 974
Plant and equipment:		
at replacement cost	5 000	
less accumulated depreciation	41	4 959
		24 933
Current assets		
Stocks	200	
Debtors	120	
Cash in hand and at bank	150	
	470	
Current liabilities		
Creditors	230	
Net current assets		240
Total assets less current liabilities		25 173
Financed by:		
Public dividend capital		12 070
Interest bearing debt		13 070
Income and expenditure account surplus		33
Total finance		25 173

Figure 4.5 NHS trust balance sheet at 30 April 19X2.

of what is contained. In practice summarized accounts are prepared with supporting schedules to give a more detailed analysis of particular figures, and each statement contains two sets of figures, one for the current year and the other the corresponding figures for the preceding year. The summarized income and expenditure account of an NHS trust is shown in Figure 4.7.

Cash, income and expenditure, and the balance sheet: a worked example

This example starts with the balance sheet from Figure 4.4 which gives the position at 1 April 19X2, the start of the financial year. Additional information is provided in the income and expenditure account for the year to 31 March 19X3. These statements are set out in Figures 4.8 and 4.9, and the number of headings has been reduced from that which would be found in practice.

	£000	£000
Income		
Health authorities	37 000	
GP fundholders	3 000	
NHS trusts	500	
Department of Health	100	40 600
Non-NHS:		
Private patients		300
Other		100
Interest receivable*		50
Total income		41 050
less:		
Expenditure (operating expenses)		
Salaries and wages	22 300	
Supplies and services:		
Clinical	5 100	
General	3 050	
Establishment (e.g. printing and stationery)	1 000	
Transport	1 000	
Premises (e.g. rates and heating)	1 000	
Agency services	1 500	
Depreciation and amortization**	4 000	
Profit (loss) on the sale of fixed assets	200	
Board members' remuneration*	100	
Interest payable**	1 000	
Auditor's remuneration*	100	
Sub-total		40 350
Surplus (deficit)		700

*   Only appears in the accounts of an NHS trust.
** Part of the capital charge for a DMU.

Figure 4.6 The income and expenditure account.

Before the receipts and payments account and closing balance sheet can be prepared, some additional information is required:

(a) During the year, £500 000 of the interest bearing debt was repaid.
(b) On 30 March 19X3, the unit received a donated piece of equipment which had cost the donor £450 000. As it was received so near the end of the financial year, no depreciation is chargeable on this asset.
(c) During the year, new buildings were erected at a cost of £1 000 000 and new equipment purchased for £295 000. Full cash settlement was made for both these amounts during the year.
(d) The land and buildings were revalued upwards by £240 000 over the year, and

	£000	Notes
Income from activities	41 000	1
Other operating income	0	1
Operating expenses	(39 350)	1
Operating surplus	1 650	2
Interest receivable	50	1
Interest payable	(1 000)	1
Surplus on ordinary activities	700	3
Extraordinary items	0	1,4
Surplus for the financial year	700	
PDC Dividends payable	(500)	5
Retained surplus for the year	200	
Retained surplus brought forward	(90)	6
Retained surplus carried forward	110	6

Notes:

1. Analyses of these figures are given in notes attached to the accounts.
2. This shows the result of performing the activity for which the entity is established, that is delivering health care. It is the difference between the income generated from this activity and the costs incurred to carry it out.
3. This is the outcome of 'normal' activities, that is the result of operating activity adjusted for the costs of financing that activity.
4. Extraordinary items are defined as material transactions which derive from events or transactions that fall outside the ordinary activities of the entity and are not expected to occur frequently or regularly. For example, the loss of a building as a result of a fire is extraordinary, and so any uninsured losses would be shown under this category. Details of each individual extraordinary item are given in the notes which accompany the accounts. Exceptional transactions, on the other hand, are those which arise from normal activities but are of such a size that they are reported by way of a note to the accounts as, without knowledge of their impact, the accounts cannot be fully understood.
5. Although the public dividend capital carries no fixed terms as regards repayment, the Secretary of State can require the trust to pay a dividend from any surplus its has made.
6. The income and expenditure account shows the surplus or deficit made during a particular accounting period. However, the balance sheet contains the accumulated result from the time when the trust was established to the accounting date. To find the amount to be entered in the balance sheet, the accumulated surplus or deficit which existed at the start of the year is aggregated with the result for the year.

Figure 4.7 Summarized income and expenditure account of an NHS trust.

	£000	£000
Fixed assets		
Land and buildings		20 000
Plant and equipment		5 000
		25 000
Current assets		
Stocks	200	
Debtors	120	
Cash in hand and at bank	50	
	370	
Current liabilities		
Creditors	230	
Net current assets		140
Total assets less current liabilities		25 140
Financed by:		
Public dividend capital		12 070
Interest bearing debt		13 070
Total finance		25 140

Figure 4.8 NHS trust balance sheet at 1 April 19X2.

the plant and equipment by £400 000. The depreciation charge in the income and expenditure account is based on the revalued amounts.

(e) At 31 March 19X3 the following balances existed:

	£000
Stock	250
Debtors	150
Creditors for supplies	290

Using the above information in conjunction with that in the income and expenditure account it is possible to prepare the receipts and payments account for the year, as shown in Figure 4.10. The difference between these two statements, as explained earlier in the chapter, is that one deals solely with cash flows while the other details the resources generated and consumed.

The outstanding balances which exist at the end of the financial year are now entered in the balance sheet, which is given in Figure 4.11.

	£000	Notes
Income from activities	31 520	1
Operating expenses	30 000	2
Operating surplus	1 520	
Interest receivable	65	
Interest payable	(720)	
Surplus on ordinary activities	865	

Notes:
1. Income:

From health authorities	27 610
From GP fundholders	3 910
	31 520

2. Expenses:

Salaries	19 000
Supplies	5 500
Other costs – paid in cash	4 500
Depreciation: Buildings	400
Equipment	600
	30 000

Figure 4.9 NHS trust income and expenditure account for the year to 31 March 19X3.

The cash flow statement

The income and expenditure account of an entity details the results of operating activity and contains transactions of a **revenue** nature. It excludes **capital** transactions such as raising a loan or purchasing a fixed asset. Capital transactions often involve significant amounts of money, and can have a critical impact on the well-being of the organization – for example, the purchase of fixed assets without the use of long-term funds is likely to result in serious liquidity problems. The cash flow statement is a relatively recent addition to the published accounts of private companies and is also required as part of the annual accounts of NHS trusts. The statement reports the sources of cash that have been raised and generated during the year and the ways in which it has been utilized. In effect, the cash flow statement contains the same information as the cash account, but standardizes the way in which the information is presented and includes a reconciliation between the net cash flow and the operating surplus or deficit.

In the statement, cash flows are divided into five main categories, for each of which a sub-total is shown:

- **Operating activities.** The cash flows which result from the 'operating activities' detailed in the income and expenditure account (Figure 4.6) are contained in this section. Therefore, it shows cash received from purchasers, and cash paid to suppliers and employees.

	£000	£000	Note
Opening balance		50	
Income	31 490		1
Interest received	65		
		31 555	
		31 605	
Salaries	19 000		
Supplies	5 490		2
Other costs	4 500		
Interest payable	720		
New buildings	1 000		
Equipment	295		
Loan repayment	500		
		31 505	
Closing balance		100	

Notes:

	£000
1. Receipts from income:	
Income generated	31 520
Add: Opening debtors	120
Less: Closing debtors	−150
Cash received	31 490
2. Payments for supplies:	
Supplies consumed	5 500
Less: Opening stock	−200
Add: Closing stock	250
Purchases	5 550
Add: Opening creditors	230
Less: Closing creditors	−290
Cash paid	5 490

The reasoning behind the calculations in notes 1 and 2 is given in Chapter 3 in the section on the relationship between cash flows and resource flows.

Figure 4.10 Receipts and payments account for the year to 31 March 19X3.

- **Returns on investments and servicing of finance.** This section contains interest and dividends paid and interest received.
- **Taxation.** This is unlikely to be of relevance to most NHS trusts as it contains the cash flows relating to taxes on revenue and capital profits.

	£000	£000	Note
Fixed assets			
Land and buildings		20 840	1
Plant and equipment		5 545	2
		26 385	
Current assets			
Stocks	250		
Debtors	150		
Cash in hand and at bank	100		
	500		
Current liabilities			
Creditors	290		
Net current assets		210	
Total assets less current liabilities		26 595	
Financed by:			
Public dividend capital		12 070	
Interest bearing debt		12 570	
		24 640	
Revaluation reserve		640	3
Donation reserve		450	4
Income and expenditure account		865	
Total finance		26 595	

Notes:

	1. Land and buildings £000	2. Plant and equipment £000
Balance at start of year	20 000	5000
Additions – purchased	1 000	295
– donated		450
Revaluation	240	400
Less: Depreciation	−400	−600
	20 840	5545

3. The revaluation reserve is the sum of the revaluations £240 000 and £400 000.
4. The donation reserve shows the source of funding of the donated assets. This will be reduced over the years at the same rate as the asset is depreciated.

Figure 4.11 NHS trust balance sheet at 31 March 19X3.

	£000	£000	Note
Operating activities			
Cash received from customers	31 490		
Cash payments to suppliers	(5 490)		
Cash paid to and on behalf of employees	(19 000)		
Other cash payments	(4 500)		
Net cash inflows from operating activities		2500	1
Returns on investments and servicing of finance			
Interest received	65		
Interest paid	(720)		
Dividends paid	0		
Net cash outflow from returns on investments and servicing of finance		(655)	
Taxation		0	
Investing activities			
Payments to acquire fixed assets	(1 295)		
Receipts from sale of fixed assets	0		
Net cash outflow from investing activities		(1295)	
Net cash inflow (outflow) before financing		550	
Financing			
New public dividend capital received	0		
New term loans	0		
New short-term loans	0		
Repayment of amounts borrowed	(500)		
Net cash inflow (outflow) from financing		(500)	
Increase (decrease in cash)		50	2

Notes:
1. Reconciliation of operating surplus to net cash inflow from operating activities:

	£000
Operating surplus	1520
Depreciation charge	1000
Increase in stocks	(50)
Increase in debtors	(30)
Increase in creditors	60
Net cash inflow from operating activities	2500

2. Changes in cash during the year:

Balance at 1 April 19X2	50
Net cash inflow	50
Balance at 31 March 19X3	100

Figure 4.12 Cash flow statement for the year to 31 March 19X3.

- **Investing activities.** Cash flows resulting from the sale and acquisition of fixed assets are included in this section.
- **Financing.** Receipts and payments of long-term funds, such as result from raising or repaying a loan, are included here.

Figure 4.12 shows the cash flow statement based on the example developed in the previous section of this chapter, especially the receipts and payments account of Figure 4.10.

The reconciliation between the operating surplus and the cash inflow from operating activities explains why these two values are not the same. The causes can be examined further by comparing the cash flows with the related entry in the income and expenditure account (I&E):

	Cash £000	I&E £000	Difference £000	Note
Receipts/income	31 490	31 520	(30)	1
Supplies	(5 490)	(5 500)	10	2
Salaries	(19 000)	(19 000)	0	
Depreciation	0	(1 000)	1000	3
Other costs	(4 500)	(4 500)	0	
Net inflow	2 500	1 520	980	

Notes:
1. The difference between cash received and income is caused by the existence of debtors at the beginning and end of the year. During the year, £120 000 was collected from opening debtors, but £150 000 remained to be collected at the end of the year. The difference between these two values is £30 000, and so cash collected was less than income by this amount.
2. The impact of 'supplies' on cash flows and costs differs because of creditors and stocks. Cash outflows have been reduced by £60 000 because creditors have increased during the year, but an increase in the level of stock required the purchase of an additional £50 000 of supplies, which used up some cash. The net effect of these two changes, £60 000 saved by increasing creditors and £50 000 spent on increasing stock, is a saving of cash to the value of £10 000.
3. The annual depreciation charge is a non-cash expense, as the cash outflow related to the acquisition of fixed assets appears in the section of the cash flow statement dealing with 'investing activities' in the year when the cash is spent. As a result, cash generated from operating activities is measured by adding the depreciation charge to the surplus, or deficit, measured in the income and expenditure account. One common mistake is to suggest that the cash inflow measured in this way can be manipulated by varying the depreciation charge; this is not possible, as a change in the depreciation charge has an equal effect on the measured surplus or deficit. For example, increasing the depreciation charge in Figure 4.9 by £100 000 to £1 100 000 would reduce the surplus on operating activities by the same amount to £1 420 000 and so the value of surplus plus depreciation remains the same at £2 520 000.

The cash flow statement takes on a particular importance for NHS trusts because of the operation of the 'external financing limit' (EFL). This is calculated for a year as:

	New loans raised
minus	Loans repaid
plus/minus	Net changes in liquid assets (cash)

The EFL is agreed every year between individual trusts and the NHS Management Executive which is responsible for the aggregate level of borrowing set within the Public Expenditure Survey. For a particular trust, the EFL may be positive, negative or zero, and will be influenced by the surplus made and retained, depreciation, proceeds from the disposal of assets, and capital expenditure plans. It can be seen that all of these elements are clearly disclosed in the statement in Figure 4.12.

Conclusion

This chapter has introduced the main accounting statements and shown how they are constructed and the values they include calculated. Anyone looking at a full set of annual accounts, for either an NHS trust or a DMU, will immediately notice that they are far more extensive than the ones dealt with here. However, this is mainly a matter of providing additional detail. In the annual accounts the main statements are summaries and occupy only a few pages, while the accompanying notes show ever more detailed breakdowns of the figures contained in the summaries. There is some additional information which must be given, such as the values of capital commitments and contingent liabilities; these items provide additional information to aid the assessment of the financial performance of the entity and, where they occur, should be accompanied by full explanations. Notwithstanding their complexity and additional material, a grasp of the techniques given in this chapter will enable the reader to understand the contents of a full set of accounts.

Questions

1. Outline the contents of the following accounting statements:

   - income and expenditure account
   - balance sheet
   - cash flow statement.

2. Explain why in the balance sheet the value of assets is equal to that of liabilities. How does an NHST obtain funds to finance its assets, and why do these funds represent a liability?
3. How is the external financing limit of an NHST calculated, and how can it be identified from the cash flow statement?
4. Why, for an NHST, is the depreciation charge a non-cash expense?
5. Both the income and expenditure account and cash flow statement report the flows of resources which have taken place during an accounting period. What are the differences between them, and which one is more indicative of the performance of the organization to which it relates?

5

Control and interpretation using financial reports

AIMS

The accounting statements considered in the previous chapter were the income and expenditure account, the balance sheet and the cash flow statement. From the point of view of management, they have a number of defects:

- They are historical as they report the financial results of activities which have already taken place.
- The information they contain is highly summarized.
- They show absolute financial values which are not placed in any comparative context.

This chapter shows how these defects are overcome in practice by:

- introducing the preparation of forecast accounts, using cash as an example;
- examining the ways in which control of working capital, especially cash, is exercised at a disaggregated level;
- explaining how accounting reports can be interpreted.

The cash forecast

Management should develop plans in advance so as to be able to decide what any cash surpluses will be used for and how any deficits are to be funded. This requires the preparation of numerical forecasts of expected cash flows, both inwards and outwards, so that any surpluses or deficits can be identified. Flows of long-term cash are likely to be irregular, while short-term flows are more regular. The procedure to convert these two types of flow into a cash forecast, taking a hospital as an example, is:

- Predict the expected amount of work which the hospital is to undertake.
- Calculate the costs related to the workload.
- Calculate the income this will produce.
- Calculate the cash flows related to the anticipated income and costs.
- Prepare a plan of the capital expenditure needed to provide the facilities necessary to generate the forecast income.
- Forecast receipts of long-term cash from such sources as the disposal of fixed assets and raising long-term loans.
- Merge all of the cash flows into a single cash forecast.

Many aspects of the cash flow forecast are interlinked. For example, some of the expected income may be reliant on undertaking capital expenditure on an asset such as an MRI scanner; if it transpires that the capital expenditure cannot be afforded, then the forecast has to be amended accordingly. Similarly, the plans must be adjusted if income and costs do not balance. Once an acceptable plan has been developed, the necessary staffing can be arranged together with the other supplies that will be needed in the short term, and the capital spending plan can be implemented.

As well as the amount of individual cash flows, it is necessary to predict their timing. The amount of detail depends on how far ahead the forecasts cover. Forecast flows for the next year may be broken down into months, while an outline plan for

	Apr £000	May £000	Jun £000	Jul £000	Aug £000	Sep £000
Receipts						
NHS contracts	2350	2350	2350	2350	2350	2350
Other income	90	90	110	110	110	120
Sale of fixed assets			500	500		
	2440	2440	2960	2960	2460	2470
Payments						
Salaries and wages	1910	1910	2000	1950	1950	1950
Non-pay items	480	490	490	500	500	510
Purchase of fixed assets			1100			
	2390	2400	3590	2450	2450	2460
Surplus (deficit)	50	40	(630)	510	10	10
Opening balance	20	70	110	(520)	(10)	0
Surplus (deficit)	50	40	(630)	510	10	10
Closing balance	70	110	(520)	(10)	0	10

Figure 5.1 Example cash flow forecast for the six months ended 30 September 19X1.

each of the next five years may be prepared on an annual basis. In general, the further into the future the forecast reaches, the less precision can be expected and so the less detail the forecasts contain. Figure 5.1 shows a monthly cash forecast of an NHS trust for a six-month period.

Some notable features of the cash forecast shown in Figure 5.1 are:

- The receipts from NHS contracts are steady, while those from other sources rise. The increase should be based on more than just optimism, especially as without the additional income a cash deficit is likely. For example, if the 'other income' stays at the April level throughout, a cash deficit of £80 000 results at the end of September.
- Spending on long-term assets exceeds receipts by £100 000. This deficit has been funded from the operating surplus, which is dependent on the increase in 'other income'.
- A possible explanation of the pattern of payments for salaries and wages is that June shows the impact of a backdated pay settlement. The increased rates then result in a higher steady level of payment from July onwards.
- The increase in non-pay spending could be due to extra costs resulting from the increased activity needed to generate the additional income, general inflationary increases in prices, or a combination of these two factors.
- The pattern of month-end balances shows growth, decline and then recovery to a small surplus. The balances at the end of April and May should be invested on a short-term basis to earn interest, while the deficits at the end of June and July could be met from a short-term source, such as an overdraft. From August onwards, a small monthly surplus is made, and will accumulate into the future if conditions do not alter.
- The size of the deficit at the end of June shows the importance of preparing a cash forecast. Arrangements must be made well in advance to cover this shortfall – leaving it to the last minute is likely to result in higher financing costs.

The position is slightly different for the parts of the NHS not organized as trusts as they are not allowed to retain surplus cash or have overdrafts. They use their superior tier, RHAs in the case of DHAs and DHAs for DMUs, as their bankers and so increase their cash drawings to cover cash deficits and reduce drawings if there is a surplus.

Once a forecast has been agreed, accounting reports of the actual cash flows for the period covered are prepared for monitoring and control. Differences between actual flows and those expected are looked into and the causes found. The results of this investigation can then be fed into the development of forecasts for subsequent periods.

It is likely that the plans will not be fulfilled in reality, and so additional resources can be bought if activity is greater than expected, subject to cash availability, or purchases and the number of employees reduced if there is a shortfall. The extent to which it is possible to adjust activity in the light of experience depends on the degree of flexibility associated with particular flows. Short-term flows, such as consumables, can be varied quickly and by small amounts, but long-term ones, such as capital expenditure on a new hospital, have to be met once the commitment to the expenditure has been made.

	£000
Stock	850
Debtors	600
Prepayments	1
Cash in hand and at bank	2
	1453
Less:	
Creditors	770
Accruals	5
Overdraft	75
	850
Working capital	603

Figure 5.2 Calculation of the value of working capital.

Working capital management

Working capital appears in the balance sheet, and is defined as the excess of current assets over current liabilities. Current assets are stock, debtors, prepayments and cash, and current liabilities are creditors, accruals and overdrafts. Figure 5.2 gives an example of how it is calculated in practice.

The balance between current assets and liabilities is of prime importance to an organization as the current assets represent amounts which will be turned into cash in the near future, while the current liabilities represent amounts of cash to be paid out soon.

Management must ensure that cash is available to pay debts at the time they fall due; to achieve this, systems are needed to control the amount tied up in current assets and make sure they are turned into cash as quickly as possible. At the same time, current liabilities should not be allowed to get out of hand as this can have undesirable consequences. For example, failure to pay creditors is likely to result in further supplies being cut off and the award of a poor credit rating. To control working capital in total requires the management of its constituent parts, and each of these is now considered separately.

Stocks

Stocks arise because there is a time lag between receiving supplies and consuming them. The value of stocks at a point in time is found by determining the quantity of each type held and then valuing it at what it cost when purchased. Where a large amount of similar items is held, or where it is not possible to identify individual units with their purchase invoice, cost is determined on the basis of an assumption, such as one of the following:

- **'First in – First out'**, often abbreviated to FIFO, values stock at its most recent purchase price on the assumption that the oldest items in stock will be used first. (The opposite approach, **'Last in – First out'**, often abbreviated to LIFO, is not met in practice.)
- **Average cost (AVCO)** calculates the average cost of items held in stock and is the method used by the supplies information system which is operated by many supplies departments.

In the balance sheet, a single figure is given for the total value of stock. In the notes which accompany the balance sheet, the total figure is broken down into three broad categories

- raw materials
- work in progress
- finished goods.

A further, more detailed, analysis is supplied with the financial returns in which the figure is analysed into such categories as provisions, staff uniforms, drugs, dressings and bedding and linen.

It is desirable, as a general rule, to minimize an organization's investment in stock, but this has to be balanced against the consequences of running out of a particular item. This conflict can be summarized as being between holding stock 'just in case' it is needed and ensuring that items are received into stock 'just in time' before they are used. While management overall is interested in the total value of resources tied up in stock, stock control must be exercised at the level of individual categories under the control of identified managers. The amount of a particular item to be held in stock is determined by its usage, the time lag between ordering it and receiving it, and any economies to be derived from buying in larger quantities.

The routine control of stock relies on the maintenance of reliable stock records. Procedures should exist to ensure that:

- all items of stock received have been properly ordered;
- all items of stock received are recorded in the stock records;
- all issues from stores are supported by a properly authorized requisition;
- the stores are physically secure and supervised;
- counts take place on a regular basis to compare the stock shown in the records with the physical stock actually held.

Debtors

Debtors represent sums of money which have been earned, but for which the related cash has not yet been received. Although, under the accruals concept, the fact that income has been earned is shown in the income and expenditure account, the cycle is not completed until cash has been received. A consequence of this time lag can be that an organization which shows a surplus of income over expenditure can nevertheless be short of cash, and so it is desirable to keep the amount of money owed by debtors to a minimum. Some of the procedures to help achieve this outcome are:

- Do not grant credit where it is not reasonably certain that the debtor is able to pay.
- Do not allow additional credit where a debtor already owes money and has not settled its debts when requested.
- Produce an aged analysis of debtors to highlight those amounts which have been outstanding longest; these can then be the target of management action.
- Ensure that invoices are issued promptly, thereby removing the excuse from the debtor that the bill has not been received.
- Monitor the amount tied up in debtors in terms of the number of weeks' revenue it represents, with the objective of minimizing it. For example, a hospital has an annual income of £52 million, which represents a weekly amount of £1 million. If debtors at the end of the year are £3 million, then, on average, debtors are taking three weeks to pay. Any growth in the credit period allowed should be investigated, and, if necessary, remedial action taken.

The value of debtors changes because:

- The volume of activity changes. If activity, and hence income, increases by 15%, then it is to be anticipated that debtors will also increase by 15%.
- The period of credit given changes. If the period of credit granted doubles from three weeks to six, then the value of debtors would double.
- A combination of these two factors. For example, in year 1 it is found that income of £78 million gave rise to debtors of £3 million, while year 2 income of £85.8 million resulted in debtors of £6.6 million. The year 2 revenue is 10% greater than that of year 1, and so, if the credit interval remained unchanged, debtors would be expected to rise by 10% to £3.3 million. Thus the volume increase explains £0.3 million of the increase. The credit interval in year 1 averages two weeks, while in year 2 it is four weeks, which accounts for the relative doubling of debtors compared with what would have resulted if the previous year's credit interval had been maintained.

In financial terms, it is a waste of resources to carry out procedures which will not be paid for. Where it is considered too risky to grant credit, it is possible to offer the alternative of payment in advance. However, despite all precautions, it is likely that some debts will prove to be 'bad'. In these circumstances, after all attempts to obtain settlement have failed, the debt is written off by removing it from the value of debtors and charging it as an expense, under the heading 'Bad debts', in the income and expenditure account.

Prepayments

Prepayments are created when cash is paid in advance of receiving the related benefit, and they often arise in the case of rental or leasing agreements. For example, when vehicles are leased on monthly terms, the agreement often requires that the cash payment for the first month is equal in value to three months' instalments; this is recovered by making no payments in the final two months. In the intervening period, a prepayment equal to two months' instalments exists, with the result that a cash outflow, recorded in the receipts and payments account at the start of the agreement, is not matched with its related economic benefit, reported in the income and expenditure account, until the end.

Management should take the impact of prepayments into account when entering into contracts for the supply of goods or services, as they tie up cash resources which, if retained, could be earning interest or, by reducing an overdraft, lessen the cost of interest payable. This exemplifies the fact that money has a 'time value', and an apparently low quote may be received because it includes accelerated payment terms. One final factor to bear in mind is that paying for anything in advance removes the sanction of non-payment if the suppliers do not carry out their side of the deal.

Cash

Cash is very much the balancing item which remains after all the cash transactions have taken place. Management's task is to ensure that the organization has sufficient cash to pay its debts as they fall due. This applies not only to the present, when sufficient cash or overdraft facilities must be possessed to pay immediate debts, but also to the future. In the latter case, amounts due in the future should be matched with the resources expected to be received in the future, and so the position is monitored using forecasts. Owing to its importance, the management of the cash balance is considered further in the next section of this chapter.

Creditors

Creditors represent amounts owed for goods and services which have already been received and are a source of short-term finance. While it can be useful to take advantage of an allowed credit period, failure to pay bills on time can have un-desirable consequences, such as acquiring a reputation as a bad payer. There can also be tangible costs where discounts are offered for prompt payment; if an organization has the cash available, then paying creditors and taking the discount can be more rewarding than using it to earn interest. The value of creditors can be monitored by relating it to 'weeks of purchases' using the same techniques as those described above for debtors.

Close control should be exercised over creditors to ensure that money is paid only to genuine ones. The control system should ensure that:

- Liability for goods and services received is only accepted where they have been ordered on an official order form. To achieve this, invoices received must be matched with order forms.
- Goods and services have actually been received. In the case of goods, records of goods received must be maintained to which the invoice is matched. A designated official must verify that services have been received before authorizing payment.
- Goods are only paid for once. This can be ensured by annotating the goods received record when it is first matched with the invoice.

Where, in operating the above controls, it is necessary to match documents, this can be achieved automatically by the use of appropriate computerized systems.

Accruals

Accruals are costs which have arisen, but for which an invoice has not been received; they often relate to items which accumulate over a period of time, such as electricity or water bills. The control of these is assisted by the creation of general cost-consciousness among staff, so that, for example, lights are turned off when not needed and taps not left running. Their value should be monitored by management, and active steps taken if they are seen to increase in an unexpected manner. Periodic reviews are also useful to establish an anticipated amount against which actual consumption can be measured.

Overdrafts

Overdrafts represent negative cash balances. They are useful to bridge short-term cash deficiencies, but are a relatively expensive form of finance. When projections show that an organization will generate surpluses over a considerable period of time, but will be short of cash, then, rather than resort to an overdraft, consideration should be given to obtaining a longer-term loan. These circumstances are likely to arise when expansion takes place, since additional stock and debtors, which have to be funded, are likely to result.

Cash management

The relationship between cash receipts, debtors and income, and cash payments, creditors and purchases was explained in Chapter 3. It is now possible to examine

Inflows	(a) £000	(b) £000	(c) £000
Income	2500	2500	2500
Plus Opening debtors	250	250	250
Less Closing debtors	−250	−350	−200
Cash received	2500	2400	2550

Outflows	(d) £000	(e) £000	(f) £000
Purchases	1750	1750	1750
Plus Opening creditors	130	130	130
Less Closing creditors	−130	−150	−120
Cash paid	1750	1730	1760

Figure 5.3 Cash management.

	Inflows		
	(a) 2500	(b) 2400	(c) 2550
(d) 1750	750	650	800
(e) 1730	770	670	820
(f) 1760	740	640	790

O u t f l o w s

Figure 5.4 Net inflows of cash (£000) based on Figure 5.3.

the consequences for cash flows of adjusting the outstanding balances by taking and allowing more or less credit, a procedure which is used as part of cash flow management. The outcome is shown in Figure 5.3.

The inflows section of Figure 5.3 shows the impact on cash received of changes in the value of closing debtors. The value of income, entered in the income and expenditure account, remains unchanged as this is the amount of work carried out, and opening debtors are an established fact. Accepting example (a) as the standard whereby opening and closing debtors are equal with the result that cash received is the same value as income, (b) shows how an increase in closing debtors reduces cash received, while a decrease in debtors as in (c) means that cash received exceeds income for the period. In practice, there is a minimum level of debtors, but the benefits of quick cash collection are obvious.

The outflows section of Figure 5.3 starts with the position in (d) where opening and closing creditors are equal, and so the cash outflows are equal in value to purchases. Position (e) shows how cash outflows are reduced by increasing closing creditors, while (f) results in cash outflows in excess of purchases because creditors have been reduced. Therefore, when cash is tight, allowing creditors to increase can provide a short-term solution. However, they must be paid eventually.

Figure 5.3 shows three possible inflows and three possible outflows of cash, each of which is determined by management decisions on the amount of credit to be granted or taken. The complexity of the process of cash management can be appreciated when it is realized that this gives nine possible net inflows of cash, as shown in Figure 5.4.

A common expression is that 'cash is tied up in stock'. Another way in which cash can be managed is to recognize this and adjust the rate at which stocks are replaced. The consumption during a period of time of items held in stock is calculated by adding purchases to opening stock and deducting closing stock. This is shown in Figure 5.5.

In this example, consumption stays the same in each of the three cases, but the impact on stock held, purchases and cash varies significantly. The three cases are now considered individually.

- **Column (a).** Purchases of £450 000 are made, which is exactly the same amount as has been consumed, and so the value of stock remains unchanged. The cash

	(a) £000	(b) £000	(c) £000
Opening stock	100	100	100
Plus Purchases	450	400	500
	550	500	600
Less Closing stock	100	50	150
Consumption	450	450	450

Figure 5.5 The impact of purchases on closing stock.

outflow may be delayed if the supplies were bought on credit, but will eventually equal £450 000.

• **Column (b).** Purchases are only £400 000, but consumption is £450 000. This means that less was bought than was used during the period, and the shortfall of £50 000 has to be made up by reducing the level of stocks held. Compared with column (a), the cash flow outwards is reduced by £50 000. Although the cash benefit of reducing stocks in this way is attractive, it must be weighed against the problems which are likely to arise if insufficient stock is held.

• **Column (c).** Purchases exceed usage by £50 000, and so the supplies acquired but not used are added to stock, which increases from £100 000 to £150 000. The cash outflow is £50 000 greater than that for case (a) and £100 000 greater than case (b).

Interpretation and performance measurement

Figure 3.1 at the start of Chapter 3 linked economic activity with the production of an accounting report to reflect that activity. Although the report represents the end of one procedure, it is also the start of another, namely the use of the report as an important input to the management process. Indeed, if an accounting report is not used once it has been prepared, then the question arises as to whether the effort and resources used to compile it have been wasted. So far, this chapter has been concerned with the underlying techniques of producing reports and the related terminology. Once a report is available, its recipients should be able not only to understand its contents, but also to interpret its implications for the organization. A number of techniques are available to help with this, some of which are of general application to all entities which report in financial terms, while others are more specific to the not-for-profit sector of the economy in which the NHS operates.

Broadly, the techniques used to interpret accounts can be divided into those dealing with position as reflected in the balance sheet, and progress as reflected in the income and expenditure account and the statement of funds. Care should be taken not to place too much emphasis on a single figure, and many of the techniques benefit when used as a basis for comparison. This can either be with the results of other entities or established standards, for the same period of time or for

	19X2 £000	19X3 £000
Fixed assets		
Land and buildings	20 000	20 840
Plant and equipment	5 000	5 545
	25 000	26 385
Current assets		
Stocks	200	250
Debtors	120	150
Cash in hand and at bank	50	100
	370	500
Current liabilities		
Creditors	230	290
Net current assets (working capital)	140	210
Total assets less current liabilities	25 140	26 595
Financed by:		
Public dividend capital	12 070	12 070
Interest bearing debt	13 070	12 570
	25 140	24 640
Revaluation reserve	0	640
Donation reserve	0	450
Income and expenditure account	0	865
Total finance	25 140	26 595

Figure 5.6 NHS trust balance sheets at 1 April 19X2 and 31 March 19X3.

	£000
Income from activities	31 520
Operating expenses	30 000
Operating surplus	1 520
Interest receivable	65
Interest payable	(720)
Surplus on ordinary activities	865
(Summary of Figure 4.9)	

Figure 5.7 NHS trust income and expenditure account for the year to 31 March 19X3.

the entity under consideration over a number of accounting periods. The former gives an idea of relative performance, and the latter allows trends to be considered.

The techniques which follow are, where possible, applied to the example developed in Chapter 4, the relevant parts of which are repeated as Figures 5.6 and 5.7.

Financial position

Analysis of the financial position looks at the structure and balance of assets and liabilities using accounting ratios. When undertaking analysis based on the balance sheet, it must be remembered that this shows the position on a single day, and can change from day to day. For example, a large amount of cash may be held on 31 March 19X2 and give a favourable impression, but this could all be spent on fixed assets on 1 April 19X2, and if the cost of the assets exceeds the amount of cash, then an overdraft will occur. The main techniques deal with working capital, liquidity and gearing.

Working capital

This measure is the value of short-term assets minus short-term liabilities, and is also known as 'net current assets'. Current liabilities are amounts that have to be paid out in the near future, and current assets provide the source of the cash to be used. Therefore, current assets should at least be equal in value to current liabilities. A negative value of working capital shows at least the need for careful planning to redress the situation, and, at worst, an organization that will be unable to pay its bills in the near future.

Further analysis can be undertaken using the working capital ratio. This measures the balance between short-term assets and liabilities, and is calculated by the following formula in which it is usual to reduce the value of current liabilities to 1:

Current assets : Current liabilities

Applying this to the values in Figure 5.6 gives:

    19X2   £370 000 : £230 000 = 1.61 : 1
    19X3   £500 000 : £290 000 = 1.72 : 1

This shows an improving trend as, at the end of the year, for every £1 to be paid out in the near future, current assets of £1.72 are possessed compared with £1.61 at the start. These are both comfortable margins as, within the current assets, cash is available for immediate payment, debtors should soon pay and provide additional cash, and the stock should, in the near future, be consumed in the course of activity and then recovered in income.

It is not possible to specify an ideal value for the ratio, although it is often suggested that it should be 2:1, but this is an ideal which is very rarely met in practice. However, some conclusions can be drawn independently of comparison with other values. If the ratio is less than 1:1 then the entity has problems as it owes more money than it is expecting to receive; the only solution is to obtain funds from such measures as selling fixed assets or raising a long-term loan. In these circumstances an overdraft is not the answer as this is included in the, already excessive, current liabilities. A ratio well in excess of 2:1 indicates the likelihood of spare resources lying idle, although this is acceptable if they are being accumulated with a view to the acquisition of fixed assets in the near future.

Liquidity

This measure is also based on current assets and liabilities, but takes a more immediate view by excluding the value of stock. This is because stock is further away, in terms of time, from being converted to cash than the other elements in current assets. It is calculated by the formula:

$$\text{Current assets} - \text{Stock} : \text{Current liabilities}$$

Applying this to the values in Figure 5.6 gives:

19X2	£370 000 − £200 000 : £230 000	= 0.74 : 1
19X3	£500 000 − £250 000 : £290 000	= 0.86 : 1

Again, there is no ideal standard, but a ratio of 1:1 shows an ability to meet short-term liabilities since they are covered by cash or near cash. The values calculated above show an improvement over the year and do not give any cause for concern as the organization will have funds generated from operating to cover the small shortfall.

Gearing

This measure is concerned with balance within the long-term sources of finance which it splits into two types: those carrying a fixed rate of interest and those which do not. The importance of this distinction lies in the fact that the fixed interest payable represents an unavoidable burden which must be met in good times and in bad, while the other type either imposes no direct cost or dividends which can be adjusted in response to conditions.

The interest bearing debt is straightforward to identify, but the non-interest bearing type needs further examination. In Figure 5.6, the sources of finance contained in the balance sheet which do not carry a fixed rate of return are:

- public dividend capital
- income and expenditure account
- revaluation reserve
- donation reserve.

These represent resources committed to the organization which are balanced by investment in assets.

There are a number of ways to derive a ratio to measure gearing, and, in the NHS context, an appropriate one is:

$$\text{Fixed interest funds} : \text{Non-interest bearing funds}$$

Applying this to the figures in Figure 5.6 gives:

	19X2 £000	19X3 £000
Interest bearing debt	13 070	12 570
Public dividend capital	12 070	12 070
Income and expenditure account	0	865
Revaluation reserve	0	640
Donation reserve	0	450
	12 070	14 025

19X2   £13 070 000 : £12 070 000 = 1.08 : 1
19X3   £12 570 000 : £14 025 000 = 0.90 : 1

These results show a decreasing reliance on fixed interest funds which has come about because:

- some loans have been repaid;
- funds have been generated from operations, as recorded in the income and expenditure account;
- increases in asset values have been matched by reserves which do not carry a fixed rate of interest.

Although some use of loans is to be expected, the general rule is that excessive reliance on them should be avoided as they carry interest, which is a fixed cost.

Financial progress

Financial progress can initially be deemed satisfactory if the income and expenditure account shows a surplus and the long-term sources of cash in the cash flow statement cover the long-term applications. Further insights can be gained by expressing costs as a percentage of revenue, as is done in Figure 5.8, which is based on the information in Figure 5.7.

The percentages, as presented in Figure 5.8, do not add very much to the raw figures, but they gain in usefulness when used on a comparative basis. For example, the balance between the two sources of income, health authorities and GP fund-holders, is likely to change over time, and the extent of reliance on either source could have implications for the certainty and stability of income. On the cost side, comparison with similar providers could reveal areas in which this one spends relatively more and so expose areas of potential saving. Over time, the cost percentages indicate how the different headings behave in response to different levels of activity; the consequences of this are dealt with in Chapter 6.

Interest cover and dividend cover are ratios which examine the ability of the concern to pay a return on the sums invested in it. These are now considered in more detail.

Interest cover

This is a useful ratio which can be used in conjunction with the gearing ratio. It calculates how many times the interest charged in the income and expenditure

	£000	%
Income:		
From health authorities	27 610	87.6
From GP fundholders	3 910	12.4
Total	31 520	100.0
Salaries	19 000	60.2
Supplies	5 500	17.5
Other costs – paid in cash	4 500	14.3
Depreciation: Buildings	400	1.3
Equipment	600	1.9
Total	30 000	95.2
Operating surplus	1 520	4.8
Interest receivable	65	0.2
Interest payable	(720)	(2.3)
Surplus on ordinary activities	865	2.7

Figure 5.8 Income and expenditure account for the year to 31 March 19X3.

account is covered by the operating surplus from which it has to be paid, and uses the formula:

$$\frac{\text{Operating surplus}}{\text{Interest charge}}$$

The result from Figure 5.8 is:

$$\frac{£1\,520\,000}{£720\,000} = 2.11$$

This shows that the operating surplus could halve and the interest could still be paid. However, if it fell by two-thirds, it would not cover the interest charge and an overall deficit would occur. A ratio of less than 1 indicates problems, and the higher the value, the less vulnerable the entity is to fluctuations in the surplus made on operating activities.

Dividend cover

This is a similar ratio and compares the dividend paid with the surplus after interest which is available to pay it:

$$\frac{\text{Surplus after interest}}{\text{Dividend}}$$

No dividend was paid in the above example, but, again, the higher the value of the cover then the less exposed dividends are to variations in the level of surplus.

Combined ratios

These measures use data from both the balance sheet and the income and expenditure account. These are considered below in more detail.

Asset turnover

This measures 'how hard the assets are working' by calculating how much income is being generated from each £1 invested in fixed assets. It is calculated as:

$$\frac{\text{Income}}{\text{Average fixed assets}}$$

Using figures from Figures 5.6 and 5.7, income is £31 520 000 and the average value of fixed assets is:

$$(£25\,000\,000 + £26\,385\,000)/2 = £25\,692\,500$$

It could be argued that the £450 000 of donated assets should be excluded from the closing value as they were acquired just before the end of the year and so had not had a chance to generate any income. If this is done, the average value of fixed assets becomes:

$$(£25\,000\,000 + £26\,385\,000 - £450\,000)/2 = £25\,467\,500$$

Using the latter figure, the rate of asset turnover is:

$$£31\,520\,000/£25\,467\,500 = 1.24$$

This figure is best assessed as part of a trend, with increases indicating greater efficiency in the use of fixed assets. One way of producing this desirable result is to dispose of fixed assets, and so managers should make sure that there are no non-productive assets.

Return on Capital Employed

This measure relates the surplus generated to the amount invested to produce it. It is of great importance to NHS trusts as it is a prime financial target, and is calculated as a percentage:

$$\frac{\text{Surplus on ordinary activities before interest} \times 100}{\text{Relevant net assets}}$$

The relevant value of net assets is found as the average value for the year of all assets less liabilities except:

- assets in the course of construction
- investments made to produce interest
- donated assets
- loans, overdrafts and public dividend capital.

In Figures 5.6 and 5.7, the surplus is £1 520 000, the opening relevant net assets are £25 140 000, and the closing net relevant assets are £26 595 000 − £450 000 = £26 145 000. Therefore, the return is:

$$\frac{£1\,520\,000 \times 100}{(£25\,140\,000 + £26\,145\,000)/2} = 5.93\%$$

The financial target has been set at 6% per year, and this has very nearly been achieved. It is likely that any shortfall will have to be balanced by greater surpluses in future, and so next year a return of around 6.07% must be aimed for.

The rate of turnover of working capital

This measure examines how long, on average, it takes to pay creditors, collect debtors and use up stocks. This is calculated by relating creditors to purchases, debtors to revenue and stocks to consumption. The calculations are preferably based on average values, and the results can be expressed in terms of days:

- Creditor turnover $= \dfrac{\text{Average creditors} \times 365}{\text{Purchases}}$

- Debtor turnover $= \dfrac{\text{Average debtors} \times 365}{\text{Income}}$

- Stock turnover $= \dfrac{\text{Average stock} \times 365}{\text{Consumption of supplies}}$

Applying figures from Figure 5.6, assuming only income from GP fundholders is subject to a delay in payment, produces the following results:

- Creditor turnover $= \dfrac{(£230\,000 + £290\,000)/2 \times 365}{£5\,490\,000} = 17.3$ days

- Debtor turnover $= \dfrac{(£120\,000 + £150\,000)/2 \times 365}{£3\,910\,000} = 12.6$ days

- Stock turnover $= \dfrac{(£200\,000 + £250\,000)/2 \times 365}{£5\,500\,000} = 14.9$ days

These results do not give any cause for concern, but they do indicate that it is unlikely that any improvement can be made in the speed of debtor collection or stock turnover. There may be the possibility of taking longer credit from suppliers, but this must be weighed against the loss of any prompt payment discounts which are currently claimed.

Economy, efficiency and effectiveness

These three measures, taken together, attempt to express the extent to which the organization is achieving its objectives.

- **Economy** looks at the inputs consumed and asks whether each of the inputs was acquired at the lowest cost commensurate with delivering an adequate service. The adequacy of the service is maintained by medical audit, and the question of lowest cost must be judged in individual cases.

- **Efficiency** is measured by relating outputs to inputs with the formula:

$$\frac{\text{Cost of inputs}}{\text{Volume of output}}$$

This gives the cost per unit of output, and relatively low figures would be deemed better than higher ones, subject to a quality threshold.

In the NHS, a number of such measures can be constructed using throughput as a proxy measure of output. For example, the average cost per patient day or case can be found, and, at a more detailed level, the average cost of each meal produced. Efficiency measures constructed in this way can be used to identify areas worthy of further investigation, but they must be used with care. For example, the average cost per case is materially influenced by case mix, and some geographical locations, such as London, have higher capital charges owing to the fact that land prices tend to be higher.

- **Effectiveness** refers to the extent to which the organization is successfully achieving its objectives. It is difficult to measure in practice as objectives are either stated in very general terms, such as 'secure an improvement in the health of the nation', or in detailed terms which may not in fact reflect the objective, like 'reduce all waiting lists to under one year'. The cost of reducing waiting lists may be to give precedence to less important cases at the expense of ones which have a greater impact in terms of delivery of health care, but happen not to have been outstanding for a year.

Summary

The use of accounts and ratios based on them as a basis for judging how well an organization is performing is enhanced if the results are used on a comparative basis. The accounts of the same organization over a number of years can be used to see whether there are any trends that can be identified; alternatively, comparisons can be made with similar undertakings to see how performance measures up to that achieved elsewhere. The latter type of comparison is known as 'benchmarking' and should be carried out against entities of similar size which carry out broadly the same type of activities. This can have significance where managers have performance related pay based, at least in part, on relative financial performance.

Conclusion

This chapter has shown how financial accounting reports can contribute to the monitoring and control aspects of financial management in the NHS. They give a useful overview using, for the most part, highly aggregated information, but the control of activity related to the delivery of patient care requires greater detail and an appreciation of the financial consequences of individual actions. These aspects are considered in the following chapters which look at financial management from the point of view of measuring and controlling costs before they are incurred, rather than reporting their impact as historical facts.

Questions

1. Outline how a cash forecast is prepared, and explain the benefits which management obtains from their regular preparation.

*2. The balance sheet of an NHS trust contains the following values at 31 March 19X5 and 19X6:

	19X5 £000	19X6 £000
Stock	900	1000
Debtors	450	300
Cash at bank	25	0
Creditors	600	750
Overdraft	0	10

What is the value of the trust's working capital? Calculate the opening and closing working capital and liquidity ratios and explain whether its working capital position has improved or deteriorated over the year.

3. An NHS trust has prepared a cash forecast which reveals a likely cash shortage in six months' time. What action can it take in respect of the elements of working capital to avoid or ameliorate this deficit?

4. To what extent do you agree with the proposition that accounting reports only provide information about the financial state of the entity to which they relate and have nothing to do with the objective of the NHS to deliver health care?

5. How can the balance sheet and income and expenditure account be used to measure the financial progress and position of an organization? Can these accounting reports be used to judge the effectiveness or efficiency with which health care has been delivered?

6

Costs and cost behaviour

AIMS

The delivery of health care incurs costs. This chapter defines costs according to how they behave in response to different levels of activity, and aims to:

- explore the meaning of the term 'cost' and examines the importance of understanding the way in which costs behave;
- analyse cost behaviour according to how costs respond to a change in the level of activity, including variable, fixed, semi-variable, stepped costs and total costs;
- apply this analysis to individual patient costs to produce a theoretical cost profile;
- examine the impact of average length of stay (ALOS) and turnover interval on patient cost.

What is a cost?

This question may sound straightforward, but the answer is not. The word 'cost' is an everyday term that most would like to believe they understand, but this confidence vanishes into an ill-defined vagueness when the exact meaning is considered or has to be explained in detail to others. Inevitably, a standardized definition needs to be agreed upon before an explanation and examination of the type and nature of costs and their behaviour can begin. Consider the following:

> Costs are measures of loss of monetary value when a resource is acquired or consumed.
>
> Perrin (1988)

This is an accountant's definition, and so further explanation is needed. The first point to note is that costs relate to **losses in monetary value** and not merely to **cash spent**, although, because the NHS has been used to operating under a cash limit system, great emphasis has been placed on cash receipts and payments. However, it is now clear that any surplus or deficit revealed by the income and expenditure account is a much wider and more representative measure of a financial performance, while the level of cash remaining is presented in the balance sheet as part of the overall financial position.

Given the above definition, to ask an accountant 'What is the cost of performing this activity?' may seem to be a question which can have only one answer. However, there are many different types of costs and many different ways of measuring them, and hence different answers may be legitimately given. Some possibilities are as follows.

- **Historical cost** measures the amount of cash paid for the resources consumed to carry out the activity. However, this ignores the fact that the value of the resources when **consumed** may be different from their cash cost when **purchased**.
- **Replacement cost** is the price of the resources consumed if they were purchased today.
- **Full cost** includes both the variable and fixed costs incurred in carrying out the activity. These terms are explained later in this chapter, and may be based on different cost bases such as historical or replacement cost.
- **Marginal cost** is the **additional** cost incurred by carrying out the activity.
- **Purchase cost** is the amount which would be paid to an external organization to carry out the activity instead of carrying it out internally. For example, the cost of having an 'in-house' catering service can be compared with tenders from private sector companies.

It can be seen that there is no single correct answer to the question posed above, as it depends on the decision the manager is trying to make. This explains why accountants can produce a range of different costs for the same activity, product or service because they can be calculated in a range of different ways. An accountant will present different figures for different purposes. This emphasizes the need to understand the underlying bases of measurement for figures presented in accounting reports.

Why study costs and cost behaviour?

The quality of any decision is based on:

- the accuracy of the information provided
- the relevance of the information provided
- the timeliness of the information provided
- the ability of the manager to analyse and interpret the information correctly.

The NHS currently is in a position whereby improvements in all of these key elements can be made, and fundamental to all of them is an appreciation of how costs **arise** and how they **behave**. Costs arise because activity is undertaken. The identification of this activity is straightforward. The ways in which the costs behave in response to changes in the rate of activity, either an increase or decrease, are more problematic.

The need to identify and measure costs and to understand cost behaviour can be illustrated by considering decision-making, which usually involves the choice over an activity:

- Should this ward be opened/closed?
- Should day case work be increased/decreased?
- Should a new consultant in orthopaedics be employed?

All of these have cost implications; either costs will rise or fall as a consequence of the decision – sometimes costs may stay the same, but usually only in the short term. The impact of changing costs is seen in the income and expenditure account, which has broadly to be kept in balance, and so the consequences of changed activity patterns must be appreciated.

The split between 'purchasers' and 'providers' of health care also highlights the need to understand costs and cost behaviour, because the contract price agreed between them is linked directly to cost. Before contract price and volume decisions are reached, managers must be aware of the costs involved, and, once the contract is in operation, costs must be controlled. Adequate control is only possible where there is a proper understanding of cost behaviour. In addition, the internal budgeting system, which is considered in a later chapter, relies heavily on knowledge of costs.

Although cost is an important factor when some decisions are made, other matters also enter into consideration, for example the clinical freedom of doctors to deal with individual patients in the manner they consider most appropriate. However, ultimately the decision to treat and the method of treatment chosen has cost implications which need to be considered in an aggregate manner.

In summary, a knowledge of costs and their behaviour is important so that the consequences of decisions can be properly appreciated.

How do costs behave?

Costs respond to changes in the level of activity whether the change is planned or not. This is important in the NHS as it is a demand-led service. Particular problems may be met with contracts which do not specify a level of activity. For example, the costs of running an Accident and Emergency unit can vary dramatically as the result of one or two unplanned incidents, such as crowd violence at a football match, a leak of toxic gases at a chemical plant, or just a frosty morning producing a large number of road traffic accidents. In the circumstances outlined, the cost pressures would not stop at the Accident and Emergency unit, as there would be consequent pressures on other areas of the hospital like the Intensive Therapy Unit.

Where the level of activity is predetermined, for example in an established contract, managers have to select methods of delivery which have an acceptable level of associated costs. The term 'level of activity' is used as it covers a wide range of possible alternatives and can be substituted for any appropriate workload measure:

- for the clinician it can mean 'patients treated'
- for the catering manager it can mean 'meals prepared'
- for the pathologist it can mean 'number of tests'

The level of activity to be undertaken and its means of delivery represent some of the most important decisions made by managers, and these decisions require some knowledge of cost behaviour.

The most direct approach to a consideration of cost behaviour is to use algebra. Some readers may not be predisposed to this mathematical approach, therefore diagrams are used to assist understanding. In using algebra, a uniform notation has developed over the years under which:

y = cost
x = the level of activity.

As the amount of cost depends on the level of activity, y is known as the **dependent** variable. The level of activity is free to vary and so x is the **independent** variable.

Variable costs

Variable costs are those that vary in proportion to levels of activity. An example is the number of drugs dispensed by the hospital pharmacy; while every patient will require a different drug regime, the volume of patients treated and a stable case mix will result in a profile of the average drug usage per patient. If no patients were treated, no drugs would be prescribed. An example is given in Table 6.1.

Graphically, variable costs can be illustrated as shown in Figure 6.1, which uses the data from Table 6.1. The linear relationship can be algebraically defined as:

$$y = bx$$

where:

y = total cost
b = variable cost
x = level of activity.

Table 6.1 Variable costs per unit of activity

	19X1	19X2
Patients treated	14 600	15 200
Cost of drugs	£365 000	£380 000
Average cost of drugs per patient	£25	£25

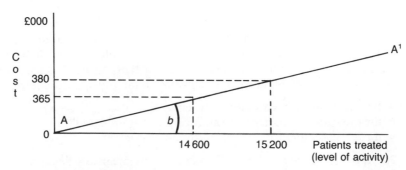

Figure 6.1 Variable costs.

Hence, from Table 6.1:

$$y = b \times x$$
$$365\,000 = 25 \times 14\,600$$
$$380\,000 = 25 \times 15\,200$$

The value of b determines the slope of the line AA^1, and, the steeper the slope of the line, then the higher is the variable cost per unit, i.e. b increases. The converse is also true so that a gentle slope indicates a low variable cost per unit.

Fixed costs

Fixed costs are those that do not vary directly with levels of activity. They stay the same irrespective of the level of activity, although they are usually only fixed up to a certain point when they will rise. Examples of fixed costs are rates, managers' salaries, domestic and cleaning, maintenance, and depreciation/capital charges. Thus, for example, in a hospital with 462 beds, whether occupancy levels are 60% or 80%, such costs are unlikely to vary. If a lower occupancy level can be planned for **in the long term** then some fixed costs may be saved by, for example, closing a ward, but these costs will remain unaltered **in the short term**.

Table 6.2 Fixed costs per unit of activity

		£000	
Fixed cost element			
Rates		140	
Management		540	
Domestic and cleaning		275	
Maintenance		125	
Capital charges		307	
Total fixed costs		1387	
Patients treated	14 600		15 200
Fixed costs	£1 387 000		£1 387 000
Average fixed cost per patient	£95.00		£91.25

The fixed cost per unit of activity is found by dividing the total fixed cost by the amount of activity and so depends on the level of activity. Table 6.2 shows that treating more patients, in the short term when fixed costs remain stable, lowers the average fixed cost per patient.

Fixed costs, using the figures in Table 6.2, are graphically portrayed in Figure 6.2. Here the algebraic representation does not contain any reference to the level of activity (x), and is:

$$y = a$$

where:

y = cost
a = constant.

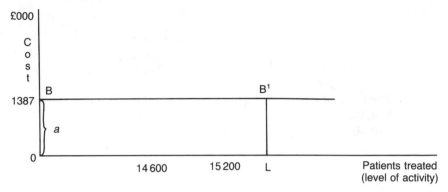

Figure 6.2 Fixed costs.

The line has no slope, i.e. $b = 0$, and the constant a, over a particular range, is determined by factors other than output. Note that the line BB[1] stops at a certain level of activity, L, above which fixed costs will rise to a new level.

Although a cost is labelled 'fixed', this does not mean that the level at which it is fixed cannot be altered. Fixed costs can be reduced by various means such as improved efficiency measures.

Semi-variable costs

Semi-variable, or mixed, costs are a third category and exhibit characteristics of both fixed and variable costs. These costs contain two components:

● one which is incurred irrespective of activity levels; and
● an element which is totally dependent on activity levels.

Common examples are telephone and fax charges, electricity and gas bills, and any other costs which have separate rental and usage components. As they have a fixed cost element, these costs also fall in terms of average cost per unit if activity levels increase.

The incremental or variable element is difficult to measure directly, but can be found by comparing the total costs of two different activity levels, as is shown in Table 6.3.

Table 6.3 Semi-variable cost per unit of activity

Patients treated:	14 600	15 200
Semi-variable cost element:	£000	£000
Telephone and fax charges	57.4	58.7
Electricity	121.6	123.5
Gas	231.5	234.3
Photocopiers	54.7	57.8
Equipment leasing	12.2	14.5
Total semi-variable costs	477.4	488.8
Average cost per patient	£32.70	£32.16

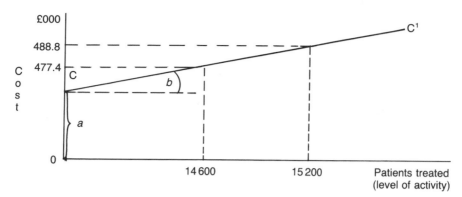

Figure 6.3 Semi-variable costs.

These semi-variable costs are displayed in Figure 6.3. The relationship can be algebraically defined as:

$$y = a + bx$$

where:

y = total cost
a = fixed cost
b = variable or usage element
x = level of activity.

The points for 14 600 and 15 200 patients treated are known, and from this the values for the fixed part and the variable element can be calculated using simultaneous equations.

At the point $x = 14\,600$, $y = 477\,400$ and at the point $x = 15\,200$, $y = 488\,000$. This provides two equations:

$$477\,400 = a + 14\,600x$$
$$488\,800 = a + 15\,200x$$

Taking one equation from the other cancels the a term:

$$11\,400 = 600x$$

Therefore:

$$x = 11\,400/600$$
$$x = 19$$

Substituting for x in either equation produces a:

$$477\,400 = a + 14\,600 \times 19$$
$$477\,400 = a + 277\,400$$
$$a = 477\,400 - 277\,400$$
$$a = 200\,000$$

or:

$$488\,800 = a + 15\,200 \times 19$$
$$488\,800 = a + 288\,800$$

$$a = 488\,800 - 288\,800$$
$$a = 200\,000$$

Therefore the semi-variable cost function is given by the equation:

$$y = 200\,000 + 19x$$

Step costs

Step costs are those which display the same characteristics as fixed costs until a given level of activity is reached. Up to a point, all fixed costs can be regarded as stepped in some way, and their identification depends on the unit of cost under consideration. For example, if the cost of a ward is being calculated, the associated capital charges represent a fixed cost irrespective of the number of patients treated. However, over the range of possible throughput of the single ward, staffing costs can be identified as stepped since increases in the number of beds and their utilization rate will, at certain intervals, require additional staff costs to be incurred. This is illustrated in Figure 6.4.

In Figure 6.4, the extra contracted cases mean that an extra ward has to be opened and the impact of this is to increase the average cost per patient treated. However, the hospital now has the capacity to treat 6240 surgery cases. To reduce the average cost to its previous level, the number of patients treated must rise to 6000, which is calculated by taking the new total ward costs of £1 600 000 and dividing it by the previous average costs per patient £266.67.

In such circumstances, it may be worthwhile considering subcontracting some cases to the private sector or another unit. Say the average ward cost per patient is

Assume that there are three 40-bed general surgery wards at a hospital treating 30 patients each per week, the average length of stay being one week. The contract for the forthcoming year is expected to be for 10% more general surgery patients treated than the 4500 cases treated last year. This raises the questions:

- Is it necessary to open another ward to meet the contractual obligations?
- What is the impact on average case costs?

Assume that a ward costs £400 000 per annum to run and that all other costs remain unchanged.

	Year 1	Year 2
Patients treated	4 500	4 950
Each ward could treat (30 × 52)		
Wards required		
		1 560
		3
		1 560
		4
Total ward costs	£1 200 000	£1 600 000
Average cost per patient	£266.67	£323.23

Figure 6.4 Step costs per unit of activity.

£300 in a neighbouring unit. If this price was charged for patients that the existing wards were unable to treat, this would result in a lowering of average costs:

Patients treated	=	4950
Wards currently treat 1560 × 3 patients	=	4680
Patients to subcontract		270

	£
Contract cost (£300 × 270)	81 000
Wards cost	1 200 000
Total costs	1 281 000

Average cost per patient (1 281 000/4950) = £258.79

The contract element represents a fixed cost which would seem to be inefficient. The average 'price' of £300 is over 12% higher than the existing ward cost per patient of £266.67. However, the use of the contractor is efficient as it keeps the average cost per patient within current levels. This is the underlying logic behind some waiting list initiatives.

The position outlined in Figure 6.4 is shown graphically in Figure 6.5. Step costs, as shown in line DD^1, are discontinuous functions and are not easy to model and even more difficult to express algebraically. They can be analysed using a technique referred to as **flexible budgeting** which is discussed in Chapter 8.

Alternatively, if the 'steps' are shallow then these costs can be approximated to variable costs. Another option can be used if activity levels can be predetermined, in which circumstances the appropriate step for the planned level of activity can be identified and treated as if it were a fixed cost. The majority of NHS costs fall into this category.

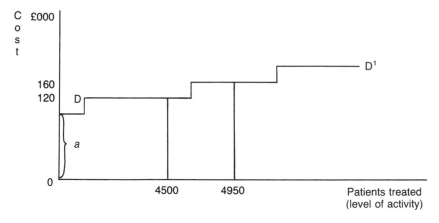

Figure 6.5 Step costs.

Total costs

Total cost is found by aggregating fixed costs, variable costs, semi-variable costs and stepped costs. In the following discussion, the stepped cost element is approximated by variable costs.

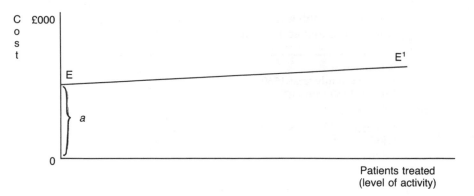

Figure 6.6 Total costs.

In the NHS the fixed cost proportion for any provider is likely to be large, with the variable/stepped element having a shallow slope as shown in Figure 6.6. This pattern of cost behaviour has significant implications for management which are discussed later in this chapter.

The line representing total costs, EE^1, is similar to the line for semi-variable costs, CC^1, examined in Figure 6.3 above. The equation for this line also takes the same algebraic form:

$$y = a + bx$$

While the total cost curve looks like the semi-variable cost curve, it is important to remember that it is an aggregation of many costs that behave differently. In particular, the rigid elements of the step costs have been 'smoothed' by being aggregated in this manner. The steps still exist, but they are far less pronounced and encompassed in the slope of the total cost line.

Profiles of patient costs over time

One of the main reasons for undertaking cost identification and measurement is to assist the decision-making process. When patient costs are considered, management decisions are based upon cost incurrence and behaviour information relating to groups of patients rather than to individuals.

A cost incurrence pattern related to time is referred to as the **cost profile**. An understanding of the 'typical' cost profile at the individual patient level is important. This is because in the contracting environment questions such as 'How much does treating 500 general surgery in-patients cost?' are being complemented by questions such as 'How much will it cost to treat one more general surgery in-patient?' The importance extends to an appreciation of the relationship of cost to the main patient throughput and output measures, such as average length of stay (ALOS) and turnover interval, that are used to assess efficient and effective use of resources.

As an illustration using in-patient activity, a patient, on admission, is allocated to a bed. Typically, it is the first few days after admission that are the most expensive. During this period a number of tests and examinations are performed and results analysed. Perhaps a surgical operation is performed, or some form of medical

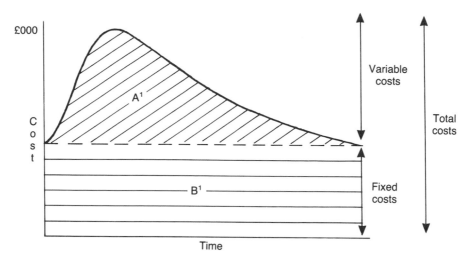

Figure 6.7 Typical in-patient cost profile.

exploration undertaken, followed by a course of antibiotics. There follows a period of recuperation on the ward, with monitoring and assistance from nursing and support staff declining as the day of discharge approaches. After discharge the vacated bed lies empty until the admission of a new patient, and the cycle starts again.

Figure 6.7 plots, at the individual patient level, the daily costs incurred over time. The fixed costs remain static as a horizontal line, while the variable costs rise to a peak early in the period of stay and tail off towards the end. The total daily cost for each patient is determined by summing the fixed and variable costs. The total cost of the stay is found by summing all daily costs, and is represented on the graph by the area beneath the curve, i.e. the sum of areas A^1 and B^1.

With a steady flow of patients the discharge of one patient is followed by the admission of the next, so the total cost of a series of patients is found by multiplying the total cost of a 'typical' patient by the number of patients in the series. However, it is not as straightforward as this because there is inevitably a small gap between the date of discharge of one patient from a bed and the admission of another to it. This gap is known as the **turnover interval**, and is measured in 'days'. During this period fixed costs continue to be incurred but, by definition, no variable costs arise. This is illustrated in Figure 6.8. The curve shown is repeated *ad infinitum* for the entire series of patients using the bed in question.

If only areas A and B are summed, whether for one or a series of patients, the costs in area C are excluded from the cost incurrence information. Ultimately, all activity is undertaken for the benefit of patients, either directly or indirectly. When considering total patient costs and associated cost profiles all costs must, again by definition, be included. Thus, the true cost of treating patient 1 in Figure 6.8 is the sum of the areas A^1, B^1 and C^1. Area C^1 must be included otherwise there is an amount of cost that is not identified against any patient.

The key variables of length of stay and turnover interval affect total cost. This is best illustrated by an example.

A general surgery ward has 30 beds, for which it is fully staffed and resourced. During a 52-week period the total number of patients treated is 1560, and the total

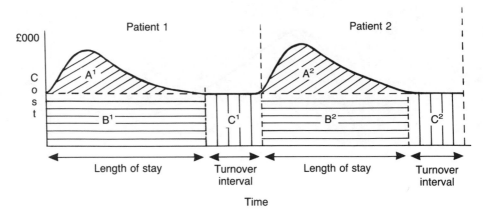

Figure 6.8 Typical in-patient cost profile series.

number of days for which this group of patients remained in hospital (patient days) is 7800. The following cost information is available:

	£
Fixed costs	520 000
Variable costs	156 000
Total	676 000

The average length of stay (ALOS) is calculated as the total number of patient days divided by the number of patients:

$$\text{ALOS} = 7800/1560 = 5 \text{ days}$$

The turnover interval is calculated as the total number of days for which beds lay vacant divided by the number of patients:

	Days
Available bed days (52 weeks × 7 days × 30 beds)	10 920
Bed days occupied (patient days)	7 800
Unused (vacant) bed days	3 120
Turnover interval (3120/1560)	2

The cost per patient is calculated by taking the total costs for the period and dividing by the number of patients:

Total costs for period	£676 000
Number of patients	1 560
Cost per patient	£433

However, this can also be calculated by considering each of the cost elements concerned.

Variable costs for period	£156 000
Number of patients	1 560
Cost per patient (a)	£100
Fixed costs	£520 000
Number of available bed days in period	10 920
Cost per day	£48
Cost per ALOS (5 days) (b)	£238
Cost of turnover interval (2 days) (c)	£95
Total cost per patient (a + b + c)	£433

This demonstrates the need to include the costs in area C in Figure 6.8 in the total patient cost calculation.

Now assume that action is taken to reduce the turnover interval from two days to one day. This results in a capability to see more patients in the same number of beds, as follows:

Total number of available bed days	10 920
ALOS and turnover interval per patient	6 days
Number of patients seen in period (10 920/6)	1820

The total cost associated with the treatment of 1820 patients is as follows:

	£	
Fixed costs	520 000	
Variable costs	182 000	(1820 @ £100)
Total cost	702 000	

The cost per patient then falls to £702 000/1820 = £386 each.

A decrease in the turnover interval reduces the cost per patient. This is because fixed costs are being spread over more patients, as illustrated in Table 6.2 above. It also increases the total cost, as variable costs are being incurred more frequently. However, purchasers may not have the additional funding available to meet these extra costs.

Assume that further action is taken to reduce the ALOS from five days to four days. The impact on costs is:

Total number of available bed days	10 920
ALOS and turnover interval per patient	5 days
Number of patients seen in period (10 920/5)	2184

The total cost associated with the treatment of 2184 patients is:

	£	
Fixed costs	520 000	
Variable costs	218 400	(2184 @ £100)
Total cost	738 400	

The cost per patient then falls to £738 400/2184 = £338.

Once again there is a fall in the cost per patient, but an overall increase in total costs. A reduction of one day each in the ALOS and the turnover interval has a marked effect on the cost per patient. In this example average cost per patient falls by more than 20%. The shorter the existing ALOS and turnover interval, the more marked is the impact of each day's reduction in them.

The actual shape of the cost profile curve varies between specialties and, in particular, at the sub-specialty or procedure level. An awareness of the cost profiles of different interventions within a specialty is of particular benefit because varying combinations of treatment needs within a patient group, known as 'case mix', can have a major impact on variable costs.

Similar principles apply to out-patient, day case and day care patients. In these cases the measure may be 'session' or 'day place' instead of bed, and time may be calculated in minutes, hours or sessions instead of days. Alternatively, in the case of out-patients and day case, the 'time' axis may be used to represent a series of visits. The shape of the cost profile curve may also be different from the in-patient curve for the same specialty, probably flatter for a series of out-patient attendances, and steeper for a day case.

Conclusion

The NHS is a very large and complex organization and the review above uses simple techniques which can only approximate what is happening in practice. However, it does provide a framework for further analysis.

One major problem that it highlights is that the majority of costs are fixed. The result is that one extra unit of activity imposes relatively little additional cost. Conversely, one less unit of activity saves very little cost. This being so, cost behaviour is best modelled in terms of stepped costs for blocks of increased activity.

It is important to understand cost profiles and behaviour patterns at as low a level as possible if these are to form the basis of managerial decision-making.

Questions

1. Why are there so many different ways of measuring cost? Is there only one right answer?
2. What do you understand by the term 'level of activity'? Why is this difficult to predict in the NHS?

3. Fixed costs can be ignored for most decision-making purposes. Discuss.
4. Why can reducing average length of stay, or the turnover interval, increase total costs?
5. Is there such a thing as an 'average' patient from the costing point of view?
*6. The finance director of the Southgate Health Trust has been asked by the chief executive to review the cost-effectiveness of a large acute medical ward which currently houses 40 beds. As a cost-saving measure, the finance director has made a recommendation that the bed number should be cut to 30 and the money saved by this measure can be used in other priority areas.

However, the costing system used to produce management information is still the same as the former unit's NHS days as no money has been found to replace it. Consequently, some of the ward's costs have been analysed over functional expenditure headings with certain costs allocated and apportioned.

		Ward Costs 19X2 £
Allocated costs		
Pay:		
Medical salaries		158 000
Nursing costs		332 000
Non-pay:		
Medical equipment		10 000
Apportioned costs and basis for apportionment		
Pharmacy	drugs issued	46 000
Pathology	test requests	12 700
Radiology	X-ray requests	18 900
Catering	patient numbers	48 700
Cleaning	floor area	25 300
Heating and light	floor area	6 400
Estate management	floor area	11 000
General management	employee numbers	50 000
		719 000

Pay costs analysis

Medical	WTE	Salary*	Nursing	WTE	Salary*
Consultants	1.00	52 000	Nursing officers	1.00	29 000
Registrars	1.00	34 000	Ward sisters	3.00	24 000
House officers	4.00	18 000	Staff nurses (RGN)	12.00	15 000
			Auxiliaries	6.00	8 500

*All salaries include employer's NI and superannuation contributions, together with any enhancements and shift allowances per WTE.

In the finance director's report, which is based on full occupancy and 52 weeks per annum, the cost saving of 10 beds or 520 patient/weeks would be £180 000.

Where do you believe the finance director has gone wrong in his estimates? Prepare a new estimate and compare your figures against the original highlighting any differences and why they have occurred.

*7. The Wenallt Hospital is a large acute DGH which manages a private patients' wing which has its own budget. The charge per day for 19X2 was £130 which covered all costs other than medical fees and theatre time where applicable. The unit has a 50% occupancy level with 24 beds, all in single rooms. The unit generated income of £569 400 during 19X2 and the following actual costs were reported:

	£	Fixed/Variable
Hotel services		
Catering	43 800	Variable
Domestic	12 000	Fixed
Laundry	8 800	Variable
Portering	8 000	Fixed
Professions allied to medicine		
Dietetics	3 200	Variable
Physiotherapy	5 700	Variable
Diagnostic services		
Radiography	9 200	Variable
Pathology	7 500	Variable
Other costs		
Pharmacy	9 400	Variable
General management	15 000	Fixed
Estate management	7 000	Fixed

For 19X3 the budget is to be uplifted by 5% for (forecast) wage awards and inflation. The rates payable on the wing were separately assessed at £40 000 and capital charges amounted to £70 000. The anticipated figures for 19X3 are £50 000 and £80 000 respectively.

Due to the layout of the ward, nursing cover is difficult to estimate. However, unlike a Nightingale ward, more staff are required when patient numbers increase. This is partly for practical reasons and partly to maintain the high standards of nursing care anticipated by the private patients. A level of one nurse cover for 24 hours a day requires five nurses to be employed. The private wing attempts to maintain a ratio of one nurse to four patients. The average salary of a bank nurse can be equated to £20 000 per annum. This is expected to be the same next year.

The patient case mix is one of non-urgent cases and can be assumed to remain unchanged from one year to another.

Required

From the information given prepare a flexed budget for both income and expenditure for 19X3 indicating whether the private wing will generate a surplus or deficit if the charge per day and occupancy level remains unchanged. Comment on the sensitivity of the budget.

7

Costs and the costing process

AIMS

The previous chapter outlined the meaning of costs, their various types and the way in which they behave. This chapter examines both the theory and the practical application of costing techniques and provides the underpinning for the processes of budgeting and pricing described in later chapters. The aims of this chapter are to:

- outline the various ways in which costs can be analysed;
- show the various ways in which elements of cost can be combined to produce aggregate costs;
- explain how costs are recorded, and the importance of a financial coding system and ledger system;
- examine the techniques of cost allocation and apportionment and why some costs have to be apportioned;
- explain how costs are measured, with particular reference to employee costs;
- examine the importance of full costing and the classification of costs between direct, indirect and overheads.

Cost analysis and costing

Costing is simply the process of determining cost. In the same way that there are many different types of cost, there are also many different costing methodologies and processes. The choice of methodology depends on the specific aim of the costing exercise and also, to some extent, the preference of the person undertaking it. This explains why accountants can produce a range of different costs for the same product or service.

However, each of the approaches and techniques is based around the same costing principles, which are themselves based upon the accounting principles and concepts. This chapter illustrates the application of these principles to a number of situations and aims to give an understanding of the 'why?' rather than just the detailed mechanics of 'how?'

Resources are acquired and consumed as part of the process of undertaking a function or activity, or producing an output, to achieve a goal or aim. Costs measure the loss of monetary value of this acquisition/consumption. Costs can therefore be expressed in three main ways:

- by reference to the input, for example the cost of:
  - a nurse
  - a pack of sutures;
- by reference to the function, which is any area or category of activity controlled by a designated manager within the overall management structure, for example the cost of:
  - a ward
  - the operating theatres
  - the district nursing service
  - the catering department;
- by reference to the output, or, more correctly, throughput, for example the cost of:
  - treating a surgical inpatient
  - a district nurse visit.

Costs calculated within each of these main descriptions can further be expressed at various levels of detail, and as various mathematical types, such as average or total. For example, depending on the basis of costing and the cost unit:

- **input costs** could include:
  - the actual cost of an identified G grade nurse
  - the average cost of a G grade nurse
  - the total cost of all nurses
  - the average cost of a nurse
  - the cost of nursing weekend overtime payments
  - the total cost of sutures
  - the cost of a specific crown car
  - the average cost of a crown car;
- **function costs** could include:
  - the cost of a particular general surgery ward
  - the cost of all wards
  - the cost of a health centre
  - the cost of all chiropody clinics
  - the total cost of theatres
  - the average cost of a theatre session
  - the total cost of the district nursing service;
- **output costs** could include:
  - the cost of a specific general surgery in-patient
  - the average cost of a general surgery in-patient
  - the total cost of all general medicine out-patients
  - the average drugs cost per patient
  - the average district nursing cost per home visit.

These examples show the need to specify clearly the **cost centre**. This can be anything from a single patient up to an entire hospital and can be defined as any activity or division for which it is deemed useful to identify the cost. Therefore, anything for which a cost is determined is, by definition, a cost centre. In all cases the basic principle of costing involves calculating input costs and then aggregating or disaggregating them and associating them with functions or activities and/or outputs. Determining the cost of any activity or output is therefore primarily a matter of determining the costs of the related inputs, that is the resources consumed.

Resources can be classified into three main types:

- staff
- assets, facilities and consumables
- information and information systems.

Under basic accounting principles it is not normal practice to put a financial value upon information and information systems and hence a monetary value can only be placed on the acquisition or consumption of the first two of these headings. Therefore, costing within the NHS almost always starts with the consideration of one or more of three sub-categories of input costs making up the first two of the above categories of resources:

- staff costs
- non-staff costs
- asset ownership costs.

One further factor to be aware of is that cost information may be required in respect of what has happened in the past (historic costs), what is happening at the moment (current costs) and what could or is anticipated to happen (future costs). Historic and current costs are factual amounts and, assuming that they have been recorded correctly and are available at the correct level of detail, form an excellent foundation upon which to construct future cost projections or against which to test them.

Cost recording

The principle of materiality dictates that there is a certain point beneath which detailed cost records are not required or are not practical. Within the NHS the level of materiality is effectively imposed because very detailed cost records have to be maintained for two important purposes.

- **Financial accounting.** By law an appropriately detailed record must be maintained so as to allow for the proper completion of the statutory annual statements of account (annual accounts). The current statements are a development of those originally introduced following implementation of the recommendations of the Körner Review of financial management in the NHS.
- **Management accounting.** Management at all levels within the NHS requires detailed information on spending levels. This information is needed both for previous accounting periods and the current accounting period and often forms the basis of extending cost projections for future accounting periods as part of the planning process.

Therefore, simply identifying total cost, although absolutely essential for determining financial performance, is not sufficient. Costs must be recorded at least at the minimum level required to meet both financial and management accounting requirements. Such detail is recorded in the financial ledger, generally known as the 'books of account', by use of a financial coding system.

Financial coding systems

The primary requirement for financial systems within the NHS is to ensure that all financial transactions are captured and recorded. This is essential to ensure that all cash spent is accounted for. Once this has been achieved, the secondary requirement is to record all financial transactions to at least the minimum detail required to comply with statutory accounting purposes. Although in terms of specific detail this minimum requirement varies from year to year, the general principle of the current Körner-style annual accounts is to identify all costs in three different dimensions:

- **On what has the money been spent?** This is known as the subjective analysis and equates to input costs.
- **Where has it been spent?** This is known as the functional, or objective, analysis and equates to function/activity costs.
- **On patients in which specialty has it been spent?** This is known as the specialty analysis and equates to output (throughput) costs.

The specific subjective, functional and specialty headings within the broad categories are determined by the Department of Health as part of the laid-down minimum requirement.

Since each financial transaction recorded must be capable of subsequent analysis into each of these three dimensions, the recording and analysis can be represented by a three-dimensional model, as shown by the cube in Figure 7.1. Each time a transaction is processed it must be allocated a financial code and recorded, or stored, in one of these code compartments.

The cube on the left of Figure 7.1 identifies the three general dimensions required within a financial coding system to comply with statutory annual accounts. Applying

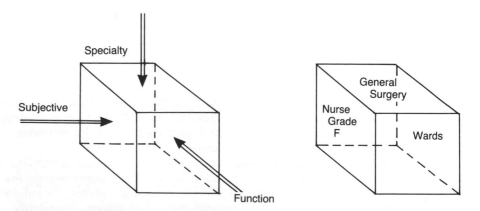

Figure 7.1 Cost accounting – the basic code box structure.

this in practice is illustrated by the cube on the right, which shows the analysis for a grade F nurse, working on a ward in the specialty of general surgery. Obviously, from whichever angle the cube is looked at, the cost at this level of detail is always the same; it is only when costs are aggregated in different ways that things can be made to appear to cost different amounts in different circumstances.

Dimension:	Subjective	Functional	Specialty
Example code:	NP10	W01	S01
Narrative:	Nurse Grade F	Ward 1	General Surgery

Figure 7.2 An example financial code.

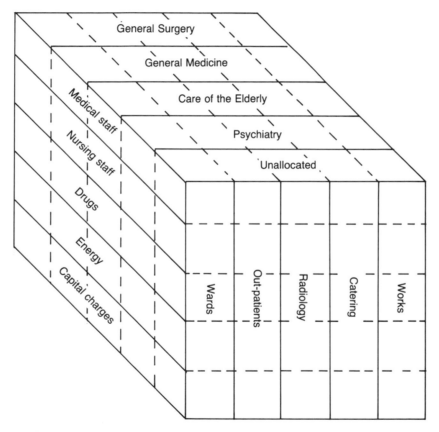

Figure 7.3 Costs in three dimensions.

The actual coding system used locally will always accommodate the three dimensions in its composition, as shown in Figure 7.2 which presents the picture in respect of only one subjective heading, one functional heading and one specialty heading. In reality things are much more complicated with hundreds of subjective codes, dozens of functional codes and dozens of specialty codes. It is when this position is reached that the true benefit of this three-dimensional approach to cost recording is realized, as is shown in Figure 7.3.

Figure 7.3 still presents a greatly over-simplified position, as it assumes the existence of only five subjective headings, five functions and five specialties. The subjective headings shown refer only to main staff groups; in practice each of these would be further divided into individual staff grades, for example nursing staff would have to be identified from grades A to I on an individual grade basis.

Figure 7.3 is equivalent to $5 \times 5 \times 5 = 125$ code boxes stacked together. If these were the only subjective, functional and specialty cost headings incurred by a provider, then this cube would represent its total running cost, and this would be true no matter which aspect the cube is examined from. However, looking at the cube from different angles provides a variety of costing information, because adding the individual compartments in the cube in different ways allows **cost analysis** to take place.

- The side of the cube has five different rows, one for each subjective heading. If all 25 compartments in the top row, that of medical staff, are added together, this gives the total cost of all medical staff employed in all functions and in all specialties. Similarly if all 25 compartments throughout the bottom row, capital charges, are added together, this provides the total cost of all capital charges in all functions in all specialties.
- The front of the cube has five columns, one for each of the five functions. Adding together all the costs in the 25 boxes of the left-hand column provides the total cost of all of the wards. The total of the 25 compartments in the right-hand column gives the total cost of the works function.
- Looking at the cube from the top, there are five segments, one for each of four specialties and one segment for temporarily storing costs that cannot be immediately recorded against a particular specialty. If the 25 boxes in the slice half way back, 'Care of the Elderly', are summed, the total cost of that specialty is found, provided that initially unallocated costs have been redistributed in an appropriate manner.

It is apparent from the construction of the cube that it is possible to identify for any subjective–function–specialty code combination the costs associated with that code. This forms the whole basis of a financial coding/cost recording system. Certain combinations never occur in practice, for example, Medical and Nursing staff would never be employed by the Works function, and Drugs would never be used in the Catering function. Such combinations are known as invalid codes and, where technology permits, the use of them is often automatically blocked in the financial ledger system.

Whilst the minimum level of code combinations is determined by the requirements of the annual accounts, it is possible to code to a greater degree of detail and then aggregate. Cost information for management purposes generally is now required at a much lower level of management and in much more detail than that required for financial accounting purposes. This has stemmed from the increased significance of financial management over the past decade, coupled with the impetus of the financial management initiatives and the improved information technology now available.

The actual level of detail is determined to some extent by local management structures and local management preferences. However, there are a number of fundamental principles. There is little doubt that an indication of the type of expenditure and the location of the expenditure is required; it is then a matter of deciding the level of detail that is needed. Locally, it may be determined that information is required at specialty or sub-specialty level, or even at DRG level or patient level. The decision as to the amount of detail to record and report must weigh up the cost of producing greater detail against the benefits derived from its availability, bearing in mind that the cost normally is an actual cash outflow, while the benefits are often more intangible and not easily assigned a financial value.

Cost allocation and apportionment

All costs, whether historic, current or future, start out as identifying spending on 'what', for example the cost of a nurse or the cost of a drug. Each cost has to be identified against the three different coding dimensions, and the level of detail at which they are recorded for each dimension is determined by the practicalities of the situation. For example, it would be impractical and costly to record actual energy usage by individual ward and department, and impossible by each patient. Even if such analysis were practical, it would result in such a multitude of code combinations being required that the financial systems would be unable to cope with them. In such instances it is usual for cost recording to take place at a fairly general level of detail and for this to be disaggregated to lower levels using averaging techniques, which can be manual or computer based. For example, heating charges may be distributed on the basis of room volumes, and, once established, the relative weights could be applied automatically by the computer in the course of routine working. This form of cost averaging is quite commonly used when deriving contract prices and wherever there is a requirement to link total costs to total activity levels.

Two terms describe the key costing techniques used: **cost allocation** and **cost apportionment**. These are, in turn, related to the main cost classifications of **direct** and **indirect/overhead** costs, which are discussed later in the chapter. Indirect and overhead costs can be apportioned in one of two main ways which are distinguished by their use, or otherwise, of activity measures.

- **Cost allocation** is used where costs can directly be identified to a cost centre. In fact, all input costs initially have to be allocated somewhere to ensure that they are accounted for. For example, the cost of a gardener can be allocated directly to the cost centre for grounds and gardens.
- **Activity-based cost apportionment** is used where costs are accumulated in one cost centre – the one supplying the resource – and are then redistributed across other cost centres – those consuming the resource – as indirect costs. The redistribution is based upon a record of each consuming cost centre's relative consumption or utilization. For example, the costs of the radiology department are initially recorded against that department and then apportioned across specialties on the basis of their level of utilization, as measured by some agreed workload unit such as weighted exposures.
- **Non-activity-based cost apportionment** is used where costs accumulated in one cost centre cannot be allocated to others on the basis of accurate workload measures, either because:
  - there is no meaningful workload measure, or
  - such record-keeping is not technically possible or is impractical.
  To illustrate both types of instance within this sub-heading:
  - management costs normally have to be apportioned across cost centres because

there is no meaningful measure that reflects the value of their relative work contribution to each cost centre;
- although an accurate record of total energy consumed by a hospital may be maintained through meter readings in the boiler house it is unlikely to be practical to meter usage on a ward-by-ward or departmental basis. Energy costs would then be apportioned, probably on the basis of heated volume.

The terms allocation and apportionment are often used carelessly in practice and are frequently interchanged or substituted. For example, 'allocation' may be replaced by 'assignment' leaving the terms 'allocation' and 'apportionment' to describe the two methods of apportionment described above. Localized terminology may present a problem until familiarity with the definitions applied can be gained. This problem with terminology is also found in the private sector.

Cost recording and time

One further requirement is that cost recording and cost identification must distinguish the period in which the cost is incurred. Periods can be as long or as short as required, but normally do not exceed a calendar year. This is essential both for management purposes to assist in performance measurement, review and planning, and also for financial accounting purposes to ensure that costs are accounted for in the correct financial year.

Past, present and future costs

The previous chapter discussed the fact that costs behave in different ways when the level of activity changes. The essential feature of cost data recorded in the financial ledgers is that it relates to information from the **past** and the **present** and is the consequence of previous managerial decisions. In making new decisions, such as on contract prices, managers can only influence the **future** and they require information on how future costs will behave. Once future costs have been estimated, control can be exercised by comparing forecast outcomes against actual results and analysing any discrepancies. This is illustrated in Figure 7.4.

In Figure 7.4, the actual observed cost X in year 1 is used to predict the forecast cost Y in year 2. In year 2, actual cost Z is monitored against Y and control exercised. X and Z form the basis for the prediction of year 3 forecast cost A, which will also take account of the experiences of previous predictive attempts, i.e. when X was used to predict Y. So if Y was based on X and proved to be 5% different from Z, then this factor can be incorporated into later prediction attempts.

Current and historic costs stored in the ledger system form the foundation of the budget control system, being used at all stages either to assist in budget setting or to undertake performance monitoring. There are many budgetary control systems operated in the NHS but they all have a number of common features, including the use of financial codes. The degree of sophistication inherent in the coding system represents the foundation of the financial information system.

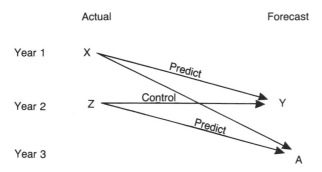

Figure 7.4 Cost prediction.

Input costs: identification and measurement

Historic and current costs for all cost headings are recorded in the financial ledgers and so are readily available. Costing past events is therefore a matter of extracting these costs from the ledger and apportioning them if required, depending upon the purpose of the exercise. It is now appropriate to consider in more detail how anticipated future costs are determined within each sub-category. Exactly the same approach applies in determining any input costs from scratch, for example where costs are required at such a low level that it is quicker to calculate them than to extract the higher level from the ledger and analyse downwards in detail.

The volume and unit cost equation

The basis of forecasting is to identify and value the relevant **volume and unit cost** equation. This involves determining how many units of a particular resource are to be consumed, and then forecasting how much each unit will cost. It can be expressed simply as follows:

$$\text{Unit volume} \times \text{Unit cost} = \text{Total cost}$$

It was stressed above that the basis of all costing involves identification of input costs, and that there are three main sub-categories:

- staff costs
- non-staff costs
- asset ownership costs.

The way in which each of these can be forecast in practice is now considered in turn:

Staff

Staff employment costs form by far the greatest proportion of the total cost of running the NHS. Generally such costs would be expected to be in the region of 75% of total revenue spend, excluding asset ownership costs, perhaps rising to as high as

80% or 90% in certain specialized services. There are many different categories of staff, and within each category there are numerous grades. However, the principle of calculating the cost of a member of staff remains the same whatever the category or grade. The terms used when identifying employee costs are as follows.

- **Basic gross cost, or basic pay,** is the amount the employee earns in a period before any allowances and enhancements.
- **Enhancements** are amounts paid over and above the basic pay in respect of additional time worked, for example overtime for night work.
- **Allowances** are amounts paid over and above the basic pay that do not relate to extra time worked. These include proficiency allowances for secretaries, on-call allowances, psychiatric lead-in payments and consultant distinction awards.
- **Total gross cost, or gross pay,** is the total amount the employee is paid for a period, including allowances and enhancements.
- **Net pay** is the amount the employee actually receives after statutory deductions.
- **Statutory deductions** are those amounts deducted from gross pay to meet any liability by the employee for income tax and for contributions to the national insurance and superannuation fund. The latter two are sometimes called 'EES contributions'.
- **Gross gross pay** is the total cost of employing the employee for the period, including employer's oncosts.
- **Employer's oncosts** are the additional amounts that have to be paid to the national insurance and superannuation funds by the employer, being additional to those of the employee. They are sometimes called 'ERS contributions'.
- **Whole time equivalent (WTE)** is a means of expressing the number of hours worked by any employee as a percentage or fraction of the number of hours worked by a full-time member of staff in that grade for the period. For example, assume that the normal full-time hours of a nurse are 35 per week and for a catering assistant they are 40. An employee working 35 hours a week as a nurse would be expressed as 1.00 WTE, but that same employee working as a catering assistant would be expressed as 0.875 WTE. It is also used to signify the staffing requirement of a department in something slightly more meaningful than hours worked; for example, a requirement for 12.71 grade D nurses to run a ward can be understood much more easily than a requirement for 445 hours of grade D work.

    WTE must not be confused with actual numbers of staff, known as the 'head-count'. A post of 1.00 WTE may be filled by a full-(whole)-timer or two 0.50 WTE part-timers, or any other combination. The term is sometimes used interchange-ably with manpower equivalent (MPE), although in some areas it may be con-sidered that there is a difference between these two measures.

When deriving the cost of an individual employee or a post it is therefore necessary to follow the calculation set out in Figure 7.5. The individual items are calculated as follows.

- **Basic pay** can be determined in two ways:
    - The **mean of scale** approach could be used. The majority of employees are paid on a pay scale, normally starting at or near the bottom of the scale, and each year receive an additional increment, i.e. an increase in salary, until they reach the top of the scale. The mean of scale cost is determined by adding together the top of scale plus the bottom of scale for that grade of staff and

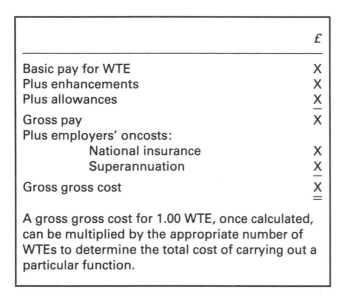

	£
Basic pay for WTE	X
Plus enhancements	X
Plus allowances	X
Gross pay	X
Plus employers' oncosts:	
National insurance	X
Superannuation	X
Gross gross cost	X

A gross gross cost for 1.00 WTE, once calculated, can be multiplied by the appropriate number of WTEs to determine the total cost of carrying out a particular function.

Figure 7.5 Calculating an employee's gross gross cost.

dividing by two. This is normally used where a post rather than a specific employee is being costed, or where a broad indication of costs is required.

— The alternative approach is to use the **actual point of scale** method. This involves identifying the actual point of the pay scale that an employee is on and calculating costs at that level, possibly allowing for additional increments during the year. This generally is the far more accurate approach, particularly where staff turnover is low, and a number of staff have reached the top of the pay scale.

When projecting anticipated future costs, depending upon the purpose of the exercise and the requirement of the recipient, the pay scales used may either be those that currently apply or, if a pay award is anticipated or due, those that are expected to apply at the time the activity will be undertaken. Adjustments for pay increases are often applied as a percentage increase to costs, derived using current pay rates, rather than costing each individual at the higher rate.

- **Enhancements and allowances** arise because a number of employees, particularly nursing and ancillary staff, may receive enhancements for evening and weekend work. Depending on the sophistication of the process required, their costs may be calculated either on an individual basis or as an average for a group of staff. Commonly a number of nursing staff are on a rota such that in different weeks they work different shifts. It may not be considered practical or advantageous to attempt to cost for each member of staff the enhancements they will earn each week. The alternative approach is to assess the average level of enhancements earned by each member of staff. This is illustrated in the example in Figure 7.6.

  The average percentage uplift of 34.57% can then be applied to each member of staff. Allowances can also be payable to certain types of staff and these have to be included in the costing exercise to ensure the accuracy of the final result.

- **Employer's oncosts** have to be added to the likely average earnings of an individual employee. There are two employer's oncosts:

Staffing requirement (WTE)	14.40
Hours per WTE	35.00
Hours required to be worked	504.00

Analysis of hours by overtime rate paid:

	Hours worked	Overtime rate	Hours paid
Basic rate	120	1.00	120
Evening rate	240	1.33	319
Weekend rate	144	1.66	239
	504		678

Average enhancement level = (678 − 504)/504 = 34.52%

Figure 7.6 Calculating enhancement levels.

	£	
Basic pay for 1 WTE	10 000	
Plus enhancements	3 457	(@ 34.57%)
Plus allowances	150	
Gross pay	13 607	
Plus employers' oncosts:		
National insurance	1 225	(sliding scale)
Superannuation	544	(@ 4%)
Gross gross cost	15 376	

Figure 7.7 Example calculation of gross gross cost.

- **National insurance** must be paid by employers as an additional sum in respect of each employee. There is a sliding scale of charges, varying with the employee's earnings, with an upper maximum amount.
- **Superannuation** is only payable by the employer if the employee pays superannuation. If an employee has opted to contribute to a superannuation scheme the employer must also make a contribution at a fixed rate.

At the end of the exercise, when all of the costs have been calculated, the result can be set out as in Figure 7.7.

Non-staff

The ease or difficulty with which accurate non-staff future cost projections can be undertaken ranges from extremely easy to incredibly difficult. The huge diversity of non-staff headings means that there is no single calculation table that can be set down to cover all situations. However, remembering the fundamental 'volume and unit cost' principle, the aim is to identify the unit of acquisition or consumption, to measure the planned level of consumption in units, and to multiply this by the anticipated unit cost.

Often a direct assessment is not possible or practical, and in such instances the techniques generally used involve an examination of past expenditure and activity profiles over a period of time. This relationship is then adjusted for non-recurring items and the effect of inflation and applied to the planned or anticipated future activity.

Asset ownership costs (capital charges)

The charge payable to represent the cost of owning assets used in the delivery of service contains two elements: interest and depreciation. The depreciation element is the sum of the depreciation charge calculated for each individual asset, and the interest charge is based on the value of assets held or, for Trusts, the amount of loans and capital. Both of these figures are generated from the capital asset register and so capital charges should be fairly straightforward to determine.

The amount of detail available depends on the manner in which the register is kept, but it should allow assets – and hence charges – to be identified in accordance with the analysis applied to other costs. The prediction of capital ownership costs is based on the existing stock of assets, adjusted for any acquisitions or disposals which are scheduled for the period under consideration.

Full costing

Costs are incurred in the NHS in undertaking a huge diversity of activities. The manner in which they are gauged and recorded is governed by the necessity to meet statutory reporting obligations and by the requirement to provide information appropriate to the needs of the management structure. Coupling this with the sheer volume of costs involved leads to a 'compartmentalized' approach to cost consideration. In practice this manifests itself in the form of functional and departmental managerial divisions and subdivisions, but with heavy operational interdependency between them. This results in a concentration by any single individual primarily only upon those costs for which he or she has been allocated responsibility within the management structure.

This rigid functional compartmentalization, which was introduced to the NHS during the mid to late 1970s, has long been recognized as hiding the true total financial costs of resource consumption decisions. A solution to this problem has been sought in a number of ways since that time. The involvement of clinical staff in the management process, and the relating of costs both to intermediate workload measures and to final output (throughput) are two particular examples.

The identification of true total costs took on new significance and seriousness with the implementation of contracting arrangements for patient care within the internal market. Now, the most important costing exercises undertaken by providers are those concerned with determining the true total, or full, costs of resource consumption decisions.

Direct, indirect and overhead costs

One further major way of classifying costs is between 'direct' and 'indirect', using these two terms in their general sense. The convention is actually to use three, rather than two classes, namely 'direct', 'indirect' and 'overhead' costs, where the latter two represent a refined categorization of non-direct cost.

Before considering definitions of these three classes in terms of costing theory, there is one very specific use of meaning to be aware of in the context of the NHS. For the purpose of completing the annual statutory financial returns, the Department of Health has set out a standard classification of all hospital and community health services expenditure, analysed between direct costs, indirect costs and overhead costs. Thus, for example, under this classification:

- direct costs include:
  - nursing and medical staff at ward level
  - diagnostic departments, such as pathology and radiology
  - operating theatres, drugs and dressings
  - professions allied to medicine such as physiotherapy and dietetics
  - other professional and technical support, such as pharmacy;
- indirect costs include:
  - medical records
  - catering
  - laundry and linen;
- overhead costs include:
  - energy
  - estates maintenance
  - management and administration
  - housekeeping
  - portering
  - ambulance and transport.

This is just one specific application of the general concept of direct and indirect cost classification. In this case it is based on the desire to impose a consistent and structured approach throughout the NHS to completion of the financial returns. The categorization has been determined by the perceived relationship of each cost heading to the **cost objective** of treating patients. The concept can, however, be applied with equal validity when considering NHS costs in other ways.

Managers are aware of the costs of resources directly managed by themselves. These are the **direct** costs of the function or department, and usually are synonymous with the budget controlled by the manager. All input costs must be identified to a function. Hence all input costs start out as a direct cost of the function to which they are allocated.

The activity of any one function frequently depends to some degree or other upon the support of a number of others. The costs incurred by these supporting functions, their direct costs, are the **non-direct** costs of the function being supported which are considered to be either indirect costs or overhead costs.

The 'rule of thumb' as to deciding whether, for a selected 'cost objective', a cost is direct, indirect or an overhead can be summarized as follows:

- input costs controlled by a manager in undertaking a quantum of workload for which the demand is directly influenced either by the manager, or by another manager, are direct costs of the management function;
- input costs not controlled by a manager in undertaking a quantum of workload for which the demand is directly influenced by the manager are indirect costs of the management function;
- input costs not controlled by a manager in undertaking a quantum of workload for which the demand is not directly influenced by the manager are overhead costs of the management function.

In practice the distinction is not so clear, and will be primarily dependent upon local management arrangements and policies, with particular reference to the level of influence by individual managers over 'the quantum of workload'. This quantum includes quality and quantity, that is the standard of work as well as the volume. One other major determinant is the meaningfulness of the actual workload measure used. A few examples will serve to illustrate these points.

- **Example 1.** A clinical director (CD) in charge of a group of wards, for example surgery, has the greatest 'influence' upon the level of workload undertaken in those wards in terms of patient throughput. This influence is exerted by the acceptance of elective admissions from the waiting list, possibly to balance emergency admissions to contract levels. The surgical CD has managerial responsibility for ensuring that the correct skill-mix of nursing staff is on duty and that nursing staff costs are controlled. These nursing staff costs are a direct cost of the directorate.
- **Example 2.** The same CD has managerial responsibility for the number of pathology tests requested by clinical staff within the directorate. The CD of the directorate of pathology has managerial responsibility for ensuring that: the correct skill-mix of medical, scientific and technical staff is available in the pathology laboratories to meet this demand; appropriate consumables are available; these staff and non-staff costs are controlled. The pathology staff and non-staff costs are a direct cost of the pathology laboratories, and these total pathology costs are an indirect cost of the surgical directorate.
- **Example 3.** The head gardener decides the type and volume of work undertaken on the gardens, including selection of staff and purchase of plants and consumables. The surgical CD, as with all other managers, has no say in determining the type of plants or the frequency of lawn mowing. All costs incurred are the direct costs of the grounds and gardens function, but are overheads to the running of the hospital and hence to the surgical wards.
- **Example 4.** The housekeeping manager is managerially responsible for the cost of employing the domestic housekeeping staff and of the cleaning materials purchased. These are direct costs of the housekeeping function. The housekeeping department cleans all the wards, including those in the surgical directorate. The surgical CD, as with all other managers, has no say in the setting of standards nor in the volume of work undertaken, i.e. floor area cleaned, each day. No record of work undertaken in cleaning each ward is maintained. The housekeeping costs are overhead costs of the directorate.
- **Example 5.** As with example 4, except that volume of work undertaken by the housekeeping staff on the surgical wards is decided by the surgical CD,

to a standard common throughout the hospital. The actual work undertaken is measured on a ward-by-ward basis using a sensible basis such as floor area. The housekeeping costs incurred are indirect costs of the directorate.

- **Example 6**. Housekeeping staff are employed on a designated ward basis and are the managerial responsibility of the surgical CD. A record is maintained of the cleaning consumables used on the ward. The CD decides the volume and standard of work which may still result in a hospital-wide standard being adopted, but this is differentiated from it being imposed. The housekeeping costs are direct costs of the directorate.

It can be noted that, depending upon local policy and arrangements, the housekeeping costs could be direct, indirect or overheads. These examples can be pursued further to emphasize the practical aspects that need to be considered in deciding the classification of a cost. Returning to example 6, assume the cleaning materials used were instead obtained from a central storeroom, their replacement being the responsibility of a 'general consumables manager', and that the record of their disposal does not identify the actual ward using them. They would then become overhead costs.

Cost allocation and apportionment

To determine the full costs of activities it is necessary to identify and add together the associated direct, indirect and overhead costs. Direct costs, by definition, are allocated to each activity and are thus capable of easy determination. Indirect and overhead costs, however, have to be redistributed between activities. The method of undertaking this dividing is termed apportionment and was highlighted earlier in the chapter.

Rather than divide costs arbitrarily, a basic tenet of financial management requires that a sensible methodology needs to be found. The most equitable approach is to calculate the division of the costs in line with the relative 'benefit' gained. An important decision, therefore, is to decide the most appropriate **apportionment basis** on which to base the calculation. There is no correct answer to the question 'what is the best apportionment basis?' in any given situation. This has to be determined locally, but should be the activity or workload measure which best reflects or influences the pattern of utilization or consumption, and hence benefit.

To illustrate, assume that the housekeeping manager is responsible for the cost of employing the domestic housekeeping staff and of the cleaning materials purchased. The housekeeping department cleans all the wards, and the function's cost is treated as an overhead cost of running each ward. This cost has to be shared among them if a more accurate cost of running each ward is to be established. Figure 7.8 presents an example calculation for this housekeeping illustration. The selected basis of apportionment of the housekeeping costs is the 'floor area' of the wards. Thus, for example, 25% of the floor area cleaned is in ward West 3 and hence 25% of the £200 000 total cost is apportioned there. This is merely simple mathematics.

In this example, and in those below, 'wards' have been used as the 'cost objective'. Exactly the same principles apply whether the cost objective is 'specialty', 'procedure', 'patient' or 'contract'. Whatever the objective, the apportionment basis decision can have a significant impact on the final outcome of the costing exercise. Consider the

A hospital has three wards, West 1, West 2 and West 3. Their floor areas are as follows:

	Floor area (m²)
West 1	450
West 2	300
West 3	250
	1000

The total cost of housekeeping for the year 19X4/X5 is £200 000.

Using 'floor area' as the basis, this is apportioned as follows:

	Cost £000	
West 1	90	(450/1000) × £200 000
West 2	60	(300/1000) × £200 000
West 3	50	(250/1000) × £200 000
	200	

Figure 7.8 Example apportionment of overhead costs.

same calculation exercise using two other bases, 'ward direct costs' and 'deaths and discharges', as presented in Figure 7.9.

The impact of this decision in terms of the variation in costs this produces is clear from the figure. Ward West 1 costs, for example, range from £25 000 to £90 000 – a 360% variation. In the case of housekeeping, apportioning cost on the basis of floor area may seem to be the most logical choice of the three. However, it may well be that in practice, for various reasons, one of the other bases is used, particularly where apportionment of overheads is involved. In fact, even floor area may not be the most appropriate choice. Perhaps some rooms require specialized cleaning or infection control treatment, meaning that some form of weighting needs to be introduced to reflect this fact.

The apportionment of overheads across activities in this way is known as **absorption costing**. Overheads are 'absorbed' by units of activity using the agreed apportionment basis, as opposed to being distributed on the basis of measured relative consumption. Where all overheads are related to activities in this manner the approach is referred to as **total absorption costing**.

Indirect costs, by their nature, are capable of being related to measured consumption and are apportioned on the basis of this measured activity. This is a form of **activity-based costing** and is a subtly different, but important, approach. To illustrate this, assume that a hospital pathology laboratory maintains accurate records of the number of tests requested on a ward-by-ward basis. Each test is allocated an 'activity unit value' using the Welsh-Canadian (WelCan) unit values, which are

A hospital has just three wards, West 1, West 2 and West 3. Their floor areas, direct running costs and number of deaths and discharges for the year 19X4/X5 are as follows:

	Floor area (m²)	Direct costs £000	Deaths and discharges
West 1	450	260	500
West 2	300	220	2400
West 3	250	320	1100
	1000	800	4000

The total cost of housekeeping for the year is £200 000.

Using each basis in turn, this is apportioned as follows:

	Cost based upon:		
	Floor area £000	Direct costs £000	Deaths and discharges £000
West 1	90	65	25
West 2	60	55	120
West 3	50	80	55
	200	200	200

Figure 7.9 Example apportionment of overhead costs using different apportionment bases.

weighted to reflect the relative complexity of each test. Figure 7.10 demonstrates two possible approaches to apportionment of the costs of the pathology function. Once again the use of different bases produces different results for each ward.

The activity-based approach tends to identify unit costs for multiplication by unit volumes in determining the amount to be apportioned rather than applying a percentage of total. One benefit of this is the extension of the concept to charge for units of activity using 'standard costs' rather than actual costs. This is explored in more detail under the topic of budgeting.

The pathology and housekeeping functions used in these examples are only two of many departments that support the running of a ward. An appropriate apportionment basis has to be determined for each of these departments. Similarly, in a large acute provider, costs may have to be apportioned across a dozen or more wards or specialties, or hundreds of procedures, rather than just the three wards used in the example. The potential for variation illustrated above is therefore magnified many times. This demonstrates why finance staff are able to produce a huge range of costs for an activity or process.

A hospital has just three wards, West 1, West 2 and West 3. The number of pathology tests requested in 19X4/X5, and the WelCan unit values of these tests, are as follows:

	Number of tests	WelCan unit values
West 1	25 000	400 000
West 2	30 000	250 000
West 3	5 000	150 000
	60 000	800 000

The total cost of pathology for the year is £480 000.

From this the cost per test/WelCan unit can be calculated:

Cost per test = 480 000/60 000 = £8.00
Cost per WelCan = 480 000/800 000 = £0.60

Using each basis in turn, the total pathology costs are apportioned as follows:

	Cost based upon:	
	Number of tests £000	WelCan unit values £000
West 1	200	240
West 2	240	150
West 3	40	90
	480	480

Figure 7.10 Example apportionment of indirect costs using different apportionment bases.

Multi-level cost apportionment

Most support functions are themselves supported by yet others. Continuing the illustration, both the pathology and housekeeping departments are reliant on other functions, for example works for maintenance, energy for heating and lighting, personnel for recruitment, and the payroll section for processing pay. The wards also rely on support from these functions.

Applying the same principles as when considering ward costs, simply taking the direct costs of, for example, housekeeping understates the true cost of that function. This, in turn, means that the apportionment of housekeeping across wards should be based on a higher cost figure to avoid understating the cost of the wards. To determine the true cost of the housekeeping function it is necessary to include an element of the costs of each of the functions that support it in proportion to the use made of them.

A further set of calculations is therefore added, with the increased possibility of cost distortion creeping in. For example, if the indirect and overhead costs apportioned to housekeeping amount to £100 000 – thereby increasing the total cost of housekeeping to £300 000 – the possible range of cost apportionment to ward West 1 is increased to £37 500–£135 000 depending upon the basis used.

Many arrangements are reciprocal: the housekeeping department cleans the pathology laboratories, the works department's offices and those of personnel and finance; the personnel function provides a service to the wards and to pathology, works and finance; finance processes the weekly and monthly pay of its own staff and staff in all other departments and wards.

Unless some structure is introduced to the process, apportionment loops manifest themselves. Consider a direct cost being apportioned from function 1 to function 2, where both functions are dependent upon the activity of the other. The apportioned costs are added to the direct costs of function 2, and the resultant total costs are apportioned back to function 1 as indirect costs. These increase the total cost of function 1 and mean an increase in the costs apportioned to function 2, thereby increasing that function's costs and increasing the charge back to function 1. This would continue *ad infinitum*. Where several interdependent functions are involved, the cost apportionment rapidly becomes very complex. Two alternative techniques can be used to overcome this.

This first of these is 'repeated distribution'. This involves use of the apportionment loop, but only for a fixed number of iterations (calculations) or down to an insignificant amount. This is illustrated in Figure 7.11.

The first apportionment could have been that of estate management rather than management and administration. This would not influence the final cost apportionment. The repeated distribution method continues until the costs have reached a relatively small level, in this case £1000, when a final apportionment is made based on approximate roundings. Computers can perform the iteration quickly and cheaply which allows for far more refinement than a manual solution.

The alternative approach is that of 'step-down' costing, of which there are two variants: 'multiple step-down' and 'single step-down'. Use of this technique involves identifying a hierarchy of functions supporting a particular cost objective, based upon their relative dependencies. Costs are apportioned in a series of steps from the functions at the top of the hierarchy through the functions at each lower level, down to the cost objective at the bottom level. This approach, which is illustrated in Figure 7.12, is not as technically complex as repeated distribution, but the multiple step-down calculations can be very time-consuming, and even confusing if costs are not tracked down through the levels. This is emphasized by the fact that, for the purpose of illustration, Figure 7.12 uses just three functions at each level, whereas in practice there would be far more.

Single step-down calculations, as illustrated in Figure 7.13, are far less time-consuming, but their ease of application must be weighed against the potential for inaccuracies when compared to the multiple step-down approach. Question 3 at the end of this chapter presents an exercise to demonstrate this.

When calculating relative percentages or activity unit costs the important principle is that, for the apportionment basis selected, only the activity units in the levels beneath the level being apportioned are included in the equation. Even though the functions on this same level may have a value for the activity unit selected this must be excluded, otherwise the calculation becomes one of repeated distribution. This is illustrated in Figure 7.14, using the same example as set out in Figure 7.11 which, by its nature, is a single step-down calculation.

Assume that in a hospital there are two specialties: general medicine and general surgery. The direct costs attributable to these specialties in 19X4/X5 are as follows:

	£000
General medicine	1030
General surgery	897

The following overhead costs require apportionment:

	£000
Management and administration	100
Estate management	380

The bases for apportionment for each specialty are:

	Employees %	Floor area %
General medicine	30	80
General surgery	50	10
Management and administration		10
Estate management	20	

Costs are to be apportioned using the following bases:

Management and administration	Employee numbers
Estate management	Floor area

Note that the service departments' employees or floor area are omitted from the basis for apportionment as appropriate – it is pointless to apportion costs back to the originating department.

	General medicine £000	General surgery £000	Management and administration £000	Estate management £000
Initial costs	1030	897	100	380
Apportion management and administration	30	50	(100)	20
			0	400
Apportion estate management	320	40	40	(400)
			40	0
Repeat: Apportion management and administration	12	20	(40)	8
			0	8
Repeat: Apportion estate management	6	1	1	(8)
			1	0
Repeat: Apportion management and administration	1	0	(1)	0
	1399	1008	0	0

Figure 7.11 Repeated distribution method of cost apportionment.

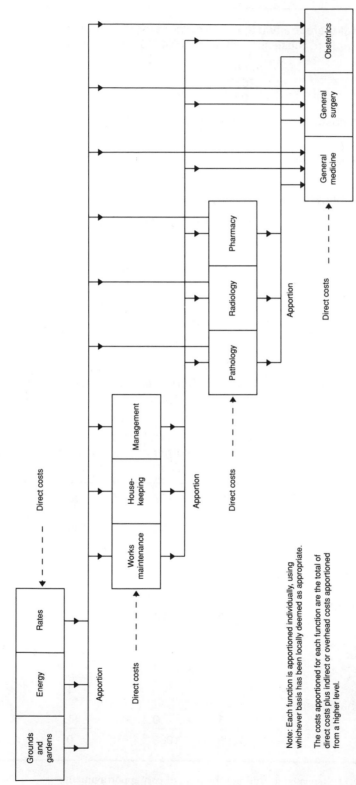

Figure 7.12 Example of a multiple step-down costing hierarchy.

Note: Each function is apportioned individually, using whichever basis has been locally deemed as appropriate.

The costs apportioned for each function are the total of direct costs plus indirect or overhead costs apportioned from a higher level.

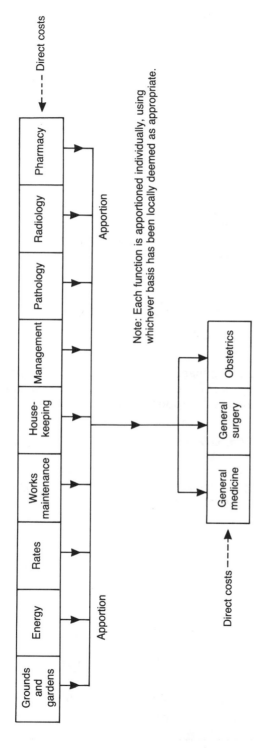

Figure 7.13 Example of a single step-down costing hierarchy.

Assume that in a hospital there are two specialties: general medicine and general surgery. The direct costs attributable to these specialties in 19X4/X5 are as follows:

	£000
General medicine	1030
General surgery	897

The following overhead costs require apportionment:

	£000
Management and administration	100
Estate management	380

The bases for apportionment for each specialty are:

	Employees %	Floor area %
General medicine	30	80
General surgery	50	10
Management and administration		10
Estate management	20	

Costs are to be apportioned using the following bases:

Management and administration	Employee numbers
Estate management	Floor area

Assuming that both estate management and management and administration are considered to lie at the same level, the percentage bases of apportionment have to be recalculated to exclude the effect of both of these functions in the apportionment calculations. The adjusted figures are as follows:

	Employees %	Floor area %
General medicine	38 (30/(30 + 50))	89 (80/(80 + 10))
General surgery	62 (50/(30 + 50))	11 (10/(80 + 10))
	100	100

The cost apportionments are:

	General medicine £000	General surgery £000	Management and administration £000	Estate management £000
Initial costs	1030	897	100	380
Apportion management and administration	38	62	(100)	0
			0	380
Apportion estate management	338	42	0	(380)
	1406	1001	0	0

Figure 7.14 Single step-down method of cost apportionment.

It can be seen that the result is similar to the repeated distribution approach. This demonstrates the balance to be accomplished between the level of accuracy achieved and the amount of effort expended in so doing. However, this is a greatly over-simplified example and in practice such similar results would not always be realized.

Classification and cost behaviour

The classification of costs between direct, indirect and overhead need not determine cost behaviour. Some direct costs are fixed or have fixed elements and some indirect costs are variable or have variable elements. However, overhead costs generally tend to be fixed when considering patient activity as the cost objective.

Apportionment bases and management behaviour

The potential for disagreement on such matters as apportionment techniques and bases leads to what is termed 'behavioural implications'. Managers have to find a variety of compromise solutions to overcome the potential disparities between bases of apportionment for indirect costs and overheads. Different methods have different advocates. The greater the proportion of total costs formed by indirect elements, then the more lively the disputes are likely to be.

The total costs do not alter if apportionment bases are changed. All that happens is that costs are distributed differently. Where this becomes particularly important is when the costing exercise has been used for contract pricing. When contracts start to be lost as well as won simply because of apportionment techniques and bases, greater attention must be placed on the methods adopted.

Marginal costing

Much of this chapter has been concerned with identifying the costs associated with an identified level of activity. These costs can be analysed between fixed, semi-variable and variable. Taken together, these equate to the total cost of that level of activity. Frequently it is necessary to identify the cost implications of changes in that level of activity at what is termed the **margin**. The principle of identifying the true total financial costs of resource consumption decisions applies equally to such changes. Indeed, such knowledge is crucial to the proper management of resources, and involves identifying the cost behaviour pattern of each of the cost elements at that level of change. The change in total cost arising from an alteration in activity level is known as a **marginal cost**. This can be positive, normally when activity increases, or negative, normally when activity decreases.

Technically, marginal costs are not the same as variable costs. If, for example, an activity increase is sufficiently large there may be step costs incurred. The marginal cost of undertaking this extra activity is the sum of the variable costs and the step costs. Nor is it correct to assume that the variable cost graph is a straight line – it could well be curved. Thus, whilst the marginal cost of one extra unit of activity may well be identical to the variable cost of the previous unit, it does not follow that the marginal cost for one hundred extra units is one hundred times greater. It is much better to remember the definition as relating to the change in total cost incurred, rather than simply thinking of any change to the variable costs element.

The derivation of accurate marginal costs in practice is dependent upon the identification of fixed, semi-variable and variable costs and their cost behaviour patterns within the likely range of activity. This work can be undertaken as part of the larger 'full costing' exercise. The development of spreadsheet-based 'cost models' is a logical means of expressing the relationships between all of these cost types and activity levels, and can form a valuable financial and business planning tool.

Conclusion

This chapter has explained how costs are identified, analysed, calculated and recorded in practice. The manner in which the initial record of each transaction is coded is of prime importance, as all subsequent analysis depends on it.

The methodologies and bases adopted when undertaking cost apportionments have a major impact on the outcome of full costing exercises, yet are an unavoidable result of the volume and complexity of functional interdependencies in the delivery of health care.

An understanding of the theory and practical application of costs and the costing process, as set out in this and the previous chapter, forms a foundation for a consideration of budgeting and pricing in the NHS. These two topics are considered in the following four chapters.

Questions

1. What are the main ways of analysing cost? What is a cost centre, and why must it be clearly defined?
2. Costs have to be recorded for two important purposes. What are these, and why are they so important?
*3. The direct costs incurred by the Northgate Health Trust in 19X5/X6 were as follows:

	£000
Medical staff	
General medicine wards	200
General surgery wards	350
Obstetrics wards	150
Nursing staff	
General medicine wards	750
General surgery wards	950
Obstetrics wards	450
Pathology	600
Radiology	450
Drugs	800
Pharmacy staff	250

Housekeeping	300
Rates	200
Energy	150
Works maintenance	180
Grounds and gardens	50
Management	170
	6000

Calculate the cost of running each of the groups of wards, and from that a cost per death/discharge, using:

(a) the single step-down method;
(b) the multiple step-down method.

The following information is also available:

	Floor area m^2	Volume m^3	Employees	Drugs issued £000	Deaths and discharges
General medicine wards	2000	7 000	60	300	1000
General surgery wards	4000	14 000	85	350	2000
Obstetrics wards	1000	3 500	45	100	1000
Pathology department	450	1 125	45	0	
Radiology department	600	1 500	40	50	
Pharmacy department	150	375	15		
Housekeeping department	30	75	30		
Works department	70	175	15		
Grounds and gardens			5		
Management department	100	250	10		
	8400	28 000	350	800	4000

8

Budgets and budgetary control

AIMS

This chapter examines the part budgets play in the planning and control process. Specifically, it aims to:

- highlight the definition of a budget, using a functional budget as an illustration;
- analyse the role of budgets as part of the planning process, together with consideration of the use of budgets in organizational **control** through the reporting of variances using feedback loops and how the variance reporting system can use managers' time effectively through management by exception techniques;
- examine the features of a good system of budgetary control;
- determine the importance of **responsibility** accounting operated through the use of cost centres;
- give an understanding of the attributes of reports such as accuracy, timeliness and the ability of managers to comprehend them;
- explain how budgets affect managerial **motivation**, why some 'slack' is necessary and how participation is the key to successful standard setting;
- consider different approaches to budgeting, including incremental budgeting and zero-based budgeting;
- discover how standard costing, flexible budgeting and a good system of variance analysis works.

Budgets and planning

A budget can be defined as:

> an economic plan relating resource acquisition or consumption to a period of time.

Three points are worth highlighting from this.

- A budget is a planning tool.
- A budget is an economic plan. This is not the same as a financial plan, i.e. one relating simply to money. Rather it is one relating to all economic resources. Budgeting therefore involves, primarily, planning resource acquisition and consumption and, only secondarily, planning money.
- Time is a fundamental factor in any budget. Thus a budget is set for a particular time period. This does not have to be a year, but budgets within the NHS are set most commonly for a financial year, with further subdivision into twelve calendar months.

Every organization has one or a number of specific plans or aims; in the case of the NHS, these are ultimately related to the overall goal of maximizing the health gain of the population. These plans are arranged according to the timescale associated with their realization, which may be:

- short term, or 'operational'
- medium term, or 'tactical'
- long term, or 'strategic'.

There are many types of budgets that are used in the NHS. Before analysing budget reports in depth it is worthwhile to present an example of a simplified functional budget which covers one month's activity (Figure 8.1). The budget columns show a budget whole time equivalent of staff employed that fall within the budget holder's responsibility. Based on this number and grade of staff, a monthly budget is calculated. This takes account of any employer's oncosts such as national insurance and superannuation contributions. The underlying computations should be sophisticated enough to isolate different pay scales and incremental points as well as incorporating any locally determined uplift factor such as performance-related pay. The actual column is produced by the financial information system which records the expenditure on each budget line for that month. The differences between the budget column and actual columns are called variances; they can be favourable or adverse.

Staff	Budget WTE	Budget month £	Actual month £	Variance £	
Consultants	7.00	25 700	32 500	6 800	(A)
Senior registrars	14.00	25 600	20 200	(5 400)	(F)
SHOs	32.00	37 700	43 200	5 500	(A)
Locums	6.50	13 500	18 200	4 700	(A)
Sub-total	59.50	102 500	114 100	11 600	(A)
Non-staff		12 400	6 100	(6 300)	(F)
Total		114 900	120 200	5 300	(A)
A = Adverse F = Favourable					

Figure 8.1 Functional budget for a clinical director.

In practice, the budget would contain more 'lines' or expenditure headings to allow for greater disaggregation of expenditure and hence enable more detailed control to be exercised. There would also be far more columns, for example showing the cumulative position for the year to date or even a forecast of the position at the end of the year based on revised figures using actual expenditure to date. The example given also provides information on the budgeted number of staff employed. Another column showing the actual number could also be included.

This functional budget is repeated for all functional managers with the aggregated provider budget not exceeding the contract income for the year. The budget lines can be updated for inflation or pay awards so long as the additional costs can be recovered under existing contracts. In addition, the budget need not be apportioned into 12 equal instalments and some degree of 'phasing' or 'profiling' can occur. For example, energy bills are higher in winter months than in summer months. It is also possible to operate a level of sophistication that accounts for the different lengths of each month, or months that have more weekends than others.

The specific expression of a provider's plans and intentions can be found in the annual business plan, which sets out the intended service delivery for the coming and future years, and, most importantly, the method by which appropriate income will be generated to meet the costs of this provision. The budget setting process is concerned primarily with reflecting the short-term, or operational, business plan in financial terms. Budgets thus represent a **formal expression** of the short-term resource acquisition and consumption plans and aspirations.

Budgets and control

In any organization, establishing goals or plans also requires the introduction of control mechanisms to ensure that the subdivisions within it act in a way that ensures achievement of these goals. Given the fact that budgets represent short-term financial plans, once established they must form part of the overall financial control mechanism. The most common and effective form of financial control is **feedback** which compares the 'actual' position at a point in time with that 'planned', or budgeted.

To realize the importance of control it is useful to take a non-financial analogy. If a long journey has to be undertaken, the first task is to establish the route that it is planned to take. Straying from this route causes the traveller to become lost – put another way, the traveller is out of control. Whoever is undertaking the journey only knows if he or she is lost by regularly observing where they are and comparing this information to the plan of where they think they should be at that time. This is feedback and without it the route prepared is of no value. If the feedback indicates that the chosen route has been strayed from, then appropriate action has to be taken to return to the planned journey.

In the NHS, the accounting system produces information on actual expenditure which is compared with planned or budgeted expenditure. The same is true for income. The differences which emerge are known as **variances** and these are analysed and reported to management, which uses them to modify activity or possibly to adjust the budget. This process is illustrated in Figure 8.2. The extent of the variance determines the person to whom it is reported. Minor variances that may even cancel out are dealt with lower down the organizational chain of

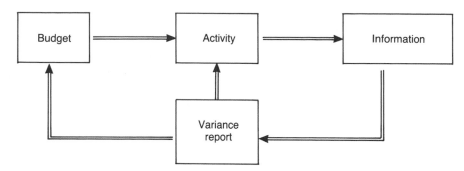

Figure 8.2 Feedback loop.

command than larger variances which may command the attention of more senior managers. This system of variance reporting is known as **management by exception**. It results in greater efficiency as senior managers do not waste their time with relatively trivial matters.

Budgets and responsibility accounting

In establishing a system of budgetary control it is worth considering the aspects that are deemed to be 'best practice'. If these features are not present then there is a strong likelihood of the control mechanism failing, or being rejected or circumvented. Rules and regulations set out by the system may be followed, but the system is seen as a 'stick' and not a 'carrot'. Ideally, managers should see the budget as a goal that they want to achieve so that the objective is **internalized**.

One way of enhancing internalization is to operate a system of **responsibility accounting**. This means acknowledging the limitations of the manager's span of control and realizing the area of the overall performance for which the manager can be held responsible. It is equally important to identify what the manager is **not** responsible for.

Most managers are responsible for **cost centres**. This means that they are only accountable for expenditure within their department and income levels are someone else's responsibility. This is typical of all functional budget holders in the NHS which is characterized by a limited degree of delegated decision-making. In the new decentralized providers there may be managers responsible for income as well as expenditure. They are involved with deciding on the pricing of their departments' services and monitoring contract performance.

A major problem which arises when trying to place only items in a manager's budget that can be controlled by that manager is the allocation of fixed overheads or the spreading of the costs of other departments, e.g. administration. While these may appear on the budget statement, no variance should be attributed to the department.

Managing through budgets

Budgets need to be managed. Otherwise there is little point in setting them. In a very small business, one person would be able to monitor its activities, and ensure that the business objectives are achieved within budget. However, in the case of even the smallest provider units and district health authorities this coordinating managerial function becomes too large for any one person and so decision-making has to be **delegated** to other managers. Such delegation extends to budget management, and budget delegation is an essential requirement in any organization, such as the NHS, where decision-making is **decentralized**.

Budget delegation requires that a designated budget manager be identified for each and every budget. Management by its nature needs to be structured if it is to succeed and managerial accountability for budget performance, as specified in the budget management structure or hierarchy, should exactly reflect the general management structure.

Theory dictates that the budget manager should be the individual who controls the level of resource consumption charged to the budget, and who takes responsibility for it. Meeting both of these requirements causes particular difficulty within the National Health Service. This is because budgeting traditionally has been based on the functional management arrangement, while spending decisions have stemmed from the actions of the clinical professions. One of the main thrusts of the formal Resource Management Initiative is to share budget responsibility in an appropriate manner between functional managers and clinical managers, in an attempt to alleviate this problem.

Functional delegation is managed via the appointment of **functional** managers, such as a hotel services manager, a principal pharmacist, a chief physiotherapist, a head of works, etc. These are responsible for the operation of their function and report on a routine basis up through the management structure.

Each functional department needs to be working to the business plan, and budgets help coordinate these interrelated functions. In the absence of a clearly defined plan and delegated management structure a phenomenon known as **sub-optimality** can result. This is where each of the functions attempts to maximize its own goals or objectives without realizing that the overall impact on the organization may be less beneficial. For example, a nurse manager may try to increase the employment of nurses at a time when the policy is to reduce staffing levels generally. This behaviour is known as **dysfunctional** and there is a tendency for it to occur in every echelon of the NHS.

Timeliness and accuracy

The budget reporting feedback loop must produce and distribute information in a 'timely' manner. The budget report must reach the responsible manager quickly enough to enable action to be taken before the next reporting cycle. For example, if the variances indicate that there is a problem with the price of supplies then the supplier can be contacted and the problem resolved before another order is placed.

The information must be accurate. Flaws in the system can result in many errors:

- expenditure may not be attributed to the correct period;

- costs may be allocated incorrectly;
- the budget not may not be flexed enough.

Even with computers mistakes are made, especially on inputting data, and the result can be a loss of confidence in the whole system of budgetary control. Whatever the cause of errors, the end result can be demotivating for managers whose performance is often measured by these budget statements.

There is a trade-off between timeliness and accuracy. In coding expenditure, mistakes can be made which result in the expenditure being specified to a temporary account or 'suspense' while the error is corrected. Perhaps the code was incorrectly recorded, incorrectly input, not specified to a budget line, etc. Expenditure items in 'error suspense' are not shown against the budget and so the reported variance is wrong, i.e. the report comparing the budget with actual results is inaccurate. So long as the amounts involved are insignificant, this is not a problem. However, the suspense account must be cleared as quickly as possible so that errors do not accumulate. This is especially true during the run up to the year end when budgets must be very tightly managed. Managers do not take kindly to corrective 'journals' appearing right at the end of the financial year possibly taking them into an over-spend situation which they are powerless to rectify.

The price of perfect accuracy, with all errors corrected prior to issuing reports, is extra preparation time. However, this may delay the reports so much that managers find them of no use in controlling their delegated functions. This is just as un-desirable as a large uncorrected error suspense. The answer lies in minimizing errors in the first place and managers appreciating the fact that some journal corrections are inevitable.

The manager must understand the report. Financially trained personnel are often accused of being insensitive to the needs of non-finance staff. The budgets must be produced in a format which the recipient is comfortable with, not in the way which the accountant finds easiest.

Motivational aspects of budgeting

Exercising control in the NHS is more about managing people than managing budgets, which should be seen in the context of how they influence people's behaviour. The main use of a budget is to monitor managerial performance and it can reflect badly on some managers. If this happens routinely, the managers may reject the budget as they never seem able to attain it. They will ignore the budget level as they are unable to meet it and perform to a level they are happy with, regardless of the wider impact on the organization.

Take the example of a laundry manager who is asked to clean 10 000 items a month, even though the laundry is capable of only dealing optimally with 8000. In attempting to increase throughout, the manager may ask employees to work overtime at enhanced rates of pay. Even with a flexed budget, this is likely to produce adverse labour variances as the standard is based on normal rates of pay. The workers may find themselves under pressure and mistakes increase. This can lead to wastage in processing laundry, e.g. machines not fully loaded, soiled linen washed with patients clothing, etc., and to adverse variances for variable overheads and supplies consumed. Meanwhile the linen manager has assumed that 10 000 items are forthcoming and will have to disappoint some wards who may now find they are faced with shortages of clean linen. The blame for all these problems is placed on the laundry manager who all the time is just trying to meet the target set. Pretty soon the manager and the workforce are likely to become very disillusioned and demotivated.

The cause of the problem was setting too high a standard. The 'ideal standard' representing the maximum level of activity may have been 10 000 items, but it does not take account of breakdowns of equipment, absenteeism due to sickness or loss of production due to delays in receiving soiled linen to wash. The 'currently attainable standard' was 8000 which may be less than perfect, but which is more representative of what can reasonably be achieved. To act as a motivating force, the budget should be set at a level just above 8000. The manager knows that the workforce can meet 8000 most of the time, but only occasionally do they process 8200. Being asked to meet 8200 may act as a motivating factor. However, the linen manager should only expect 8000 items as the higher level of 8200 may not be achieved. This realistic approach to budget setting also, in this example, reveals at an early stage the likelihood that alternative arrangements must be made for the 2000 items expected in excess of the 8000 which the laundry can handle.

This shows the importance of **participation** in budget setting. The person best placed to decide the budget standard was the manager being controlled by the budget, and this is usually the case. However, it seems somewhat perverse to allow the manager to decide the budget level, as a low standard may be selected. There is a need for benchmarks and comparisons with other similar departments to ensure that any material bias is avoided. Participation is vital if acceptance of the budget is to be achieved. It is easy to see that participation can lead to bias and 'slack' being introduced so that managers know they are able to meet the standard set. The laundry manager in the example would like the budget set at 7500 items, but this would not stretch the department at all and therefore would be less cost-effective. Through careful examination of previous records, bias introduction can be reduced and if the reward system is structured appropriately, for example paying managers and workers a bonus for reaching peak performance, then the budget can be set at a relatively high level.

'Slack' can be tolerated in budget level setting as a means of reducing conflict between different departments. However, management needs to be wary of 'empire building' and must monitor consistently overstated funding requests which allow slack to build up to unjustifiable levels. This is especially true of the NHS where managers are to some extent protected from market forces and often benefit from the effects of incremental budgeting (discussed below).

Basic approaches to budgeting

The practical aspects of budgeting and budget calculation methodologies are examined in detail in the following chapter. At this point it is only necessary to consider the theoretical aspects of the main approaches to budget setting used in the NHS.

- **Incremental budgeting** has always been used extensively throughout the NHS, and indeed throughout the public sector. It involves starting with last year's budget and concentrating on adjusting it to reflect known changes between the two years. This requires taking account of inflation and pay awards as well as any changes in service provision and activity levels. This method of budgeting has the advantage of being relatively cheap to administer and easy for non-financial managers to understand.

- **Zero-based budgeting (ZBB)** starts with the assumption that budget managers will receive zero resources and requires the desired level of expenditure to be justified each time. This is a costly alternative to administer, but it can produce savings by eliminating built-up 'slack'. It is therefore worthwhile attempting a ZBB exercise every few years.

Under either approach there is an assumption about the level of activity to be provided from within the budget. Once set, such budgets may be considered as **fixed** for the year, subject to any agreed adjustments arising from pre-planned changes to the level or manner of services provided during the year. Changes in activity levels will not automatically result in changes to the budgeted funding. Alternatively, the budget-setting policy may be that the budget funding will automatically be **flexed** to reflect the actual activity levels.

Standard costing and flexible budgeting

Many providers are moving to a more advanced system of budgeting known as flexible budgeting, which is itself a form of what is termed **standard costing**. This is a technique which uses standards for costs and income for the purpose of control through variance analysis.

The standard cost for an expense item can be determined in many ways. The use of 'ideal' standards can be dysfunctional as was the case with the laundry manager above. It is more likely that historic cost information will be used to prepare the standard cost, with adjustments for changes in circumstances and, say, efficiency savings. The established standard needs to be reviewed regularly.

A budget is based on forecasts of activity that may not be realized in the fullness of time. It is therefore unfair to penalize managers if, for example, activity has been increased because more patients than contracted for have been seen due to a high incidence of emergencies, or the purchasing authority has changed the specification of one or more of its contracts. If activity has been higher than budgeted, then the costs associated with that activity level will be higher, and vice versa. The budget is therefore adjusted, i.e. flexed, for the volume of activity.

The impact this flexing can have on understanding and interpreting budget performance is shown in the following two illustrations. First, Figure 8.3 presents the position where budgets are not flexed to reflect changes in activity levels. The standards for each budget line have already been set and agreed. So the £2 per patient day for staffing, for example, may have been derived by taking last year's expenditure on staff and dividing it by the number of patient days for the same period.

From the unflexed budget in Figure 8.3 the catering manager is faced with a number of favourable variances, indicated by the 'F' next to the difference between the budgeted expenditure and the actual expenditure. On the face of it the budget is £2250 underspent and the catering manager should be commended. However, the budget has been set on the assumption that meals for 10 000 patient days will be

	Budgeted	Actual	Variance
Patient days	10 000	8 000	
	£	£	£
Staff (£2/patient day)	20 000	19 500	500 F
Provisions (£1/patient day)	10 000	9 250	750 F
Variable overheads (£0.5/patient day)	5 000	4 000	1000 F
Fixed overheads	7 000	7 000	
	42 000	39 750	2250 F

Figure 8.3 Unflexed budget for a catering department.

	Budgeted	Actual	Variance
Patient days	8 000	8 000	
	£	£	£
Staff (£2/patient day)	16 000	19 500	3500 A
Provisions (£1/patient day)	8 000	9 250	1250 A
Variable overheads (£0.5/patient day)	4 000	4 000	–
Fixed overheads	7 000	7 000	–
	35 000	39 750	4750 A

Figure 8.4 Flexed budget for a catering department.

produced. In the above analysis the **volume variance** has not been accounted for and the budgeted level needs to be adjusted for the lower level of activity.

Now consider Figure 8.4, which presents the same situation but with budgets flexed to reflect the volume variance. Note how the 'budgeted activity' has been reduced to the level of actual activity, i.e. 8000 patient days. The 'staff', 'provisions' and 'variable overheads' lines now reflect the costs that should be incurred to provide that lower number of meals. When compared to the actual costs this flexed budget indicates that the catering manager has overspent the budget on staff and provisions producing an adverse, i.e. unfavourable, variance, 'A'. Flexing the budget has identified problems in respect of the staff costs and the provisions costs. Using standard costing techniques, the reasons for the variances on these two heads can be determined and the appropriate action taken.

The fixed costs, if budgeted accurately, remain the same regardless of the activity level.

Variance analysis

The variance produced under a flexible budgeting system can be divided into two components. These are the **price (or rate) variance** and the **usage/volume (or efficiency) variance**. A price variance measures the difference between the amount the department expected to pay for the resource and the amount actually paid. The usage variance measures the difference between the quantity of a resource the department expected to use and the amount actually used.

Variances can be thought of graphically as in Figure 8.5. The budget is the area represented by the rectangle enclosed in bold lines, SP × SQ. The abbreviations refer to the terms standard price and standard quantity. The actual expenditure is given by the rectangle enclosed in thin lines, AP × AQ. This refers to actual price times the actual quantity.

The following formulae can be used to calculate the variances:

Price variance: AQ × (SP − AP)
Usage variance: SP × (SQ − AQ)

Figure 8.6 provides a practical example. The efficiency and usage variances amount to (£200 + £100) = £300 (A) and have been caused by the extra X-ray films used over and above the standard set for the month. The radiology manager cannot be held responsible for this unless the radiographers have wasted films through inefficient procedures, e.g. poor positioning of patients resulting in abortive exposures. Assuming no wasted exposures, the main reason for this variance is likely to be the number of requests for X-rays made by clinicians. If adequate records are kept then this variance can be apportioned amongst the clinical directorates.

The staff rate variance of £60 (F) is the responsibility of the radiology manager and requires further investigation. It could be caused either by paying radiographers at a lower hourly rate than anticipated which is unlikely, or by taking less time than planned to take the exposures, or by using staff at a lower than anticipated grade – and hence hourly rate – to perform some of the work.

The price variance of £120 (adverse) on the non-staff budget line is caused by 1200 films being used at a price of £0.10 more than standard. This is the responsibility of the supplies manager, who has paid more for the films than the standard rate. As a consequence this variance can be allocated accordingly.

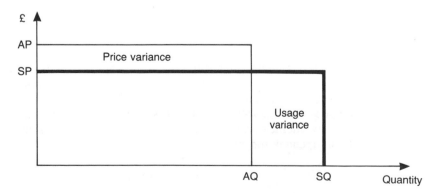

Figure 8.5 Variance analysis.

> The radiology department manager has a budget set on just two budget lines, staff and non-staff. The performance over the month shows an adverse variance, but who is responsible?
>
> | | SP per film £ | SQ films | Budget £ | AP per film £ | AQ films | Actual £ | Variance £ |
> |---|---|---|---|---|---|---|---|
> | Staff | 1.00 | 1000 | 1000 | 0.95 | 1200 | 1140 | 140 A |
> | Non-Staff | 0.50 | 1000 | 500 | 0.60 | 1200 | 720 | 220 A |
> | | | | 1500 | | | 1860 | 360 A |
>
> | | | | £ | Responsible manager |
> |---|---|---|---|---|
> | *Staff variances:* | | | | |
> | Rate: | 1200 × (1.00 − 0.95) | = | 60 F | Radiologist |
> | Efficiency: | 1.00 × (1000 − 1200) | = | 200 A | Clinician |
> | | | | 140 A | |
> | | | | | |
> | *Non-staff variances:* | | | | |
> | | | | £ | |
> | Price: | 1200 × (0.5 − 0.60) | = | 120 A | Supplies |
> | Usage: | 0.50 × (1000 − 1200) | = | 100 A | Clinician |
> | | | | 220 A | |
> | Total variance (140 + 220) | | | 360 A | |

Figure 8.6 Variance analysis in a radiology department.

So, far from being reprimanded for poor performance, the radiology manager is to be congratulated for the £60 favourable variance. The supplies manager and the clinicians have caused the remaining adverse variance of £420. Even the usage/efficiency variance may not be a problem if it has been caused by additional patients being seen and is covered by additional income.

Variances often are interdependent. If the supplies manager obtains cheap films, a favourable variance can be produced for the supplies department. However, the knock-on effect may be that the films purchased are of an inferior quality than the standard films. As a consequence, the radiographers may have poorer results causing an increase in the number of necessary exposures. The result is an adverse variance attributable to the radiology manager. If the total variance is adverse this can be sub-optimal. If the total variance is favourable then the standards should be adjusted to reflect the new circumstances.

It is important to realize that variances can be caused by incorrect standards as much as by inefficiencies in operations, and for this reason standards must constantly be updated and monitored.

Conclusion

An organization cannot be controlled without adhering to a plan. Budgets represent plans in financial terms for managers to use to exercise control. The comparison of actual results with the plan indicates divergences known as variances which can be analysed and the causes identified. It is important for mangers to be involved in the system of budgetary control and to participate in standard setting. This increases motivation and ensures that the system of budgetary control operates effectively.

Questions

1. Why is it necessary to have a plan in order to control an organization? Surely 'doing the same as last year' is as good a strategy as any?
2. 'There is no such thing as a standard cost in the NHS. All providers are different and so are all patients. You may as well leave the theory where it is and concentrate on what works in practice.' Is there any substance to the sentiments expressed by this disenchanted manager?
3. 'Variance analysis is demotivational because it is a system that merely apportions blame and does not provide solutions to problems.' Discuss.
4. 'It is no good trying to plan too far ahead as circumstances change so quickly. Even planning for one year is foolhardy and a waste of valuable time and money.' How far do you agree or disagree with this statement?
*5. The pathology department manager has a budget set on just two budget lines, staff and non-staff. The performance over the month shows a favourable variance, but should the pathology manager be congratulated?

	SP £	SQ tests	Budget £	AP £	AQ tests	Actual £	Variance £
Staff	1.50	2500	3750	1.75	2400	4200	450 A
Non-Staff	1.00	2500	2500	0.80	2400	1920	580 F
			6250			6120	130 F

9

The budgeting process

AIMS

The previous chapter examined the part budgets play in the process of planning and control, and considered different approaches to budgeting, including flexible budgeting and variance analysis. This chapter extends these discussions, applying them to the NHS budgeting process. In particular it:

- identifies the fundamental resource planning rule;
- examines the budget setting process, identifying the major types of budget;
- illustrates the practical benefits of variance analysis;
- explains the importance of achieving a balanced budget strategy, and the means by which this is accomplished;
- discusses the advantages and potential pitfalls of the 'fixed' and 'flexible' approaches to budgeting.

Budgets and financial control

A budget is a tool used to relate planned resource acquisition and consumption to a period of time. Financial control can only be maintained if resource consumption is expressed in cost terms and is properly planned and budgeted. Thus, budgets can be thought of as **planned costs**. Plans should not be made to incur a cost unless an adequate budget is available against which to charge it; this means that all planned costs have to be represented by equivalent budgets. The following fundamental rule, referred to as the 'budgets equals costs' rule, is therefore applicable when considering resource consumption plans:

Total budget = Total planned cost

All budgets and all planned costs are the responsibility of an identified individual, and so all resources – staff, assets and consumables – must be controlled by a designated budget manager. The manager's role cannot be underestimated, because the control of budget performance requires a full awareness of the content of the budget and its method of calculation, and of the associated resource consumption behaviour patterns.

Prior to contracting, it was only necessary to create budgets for revenue expenditure (plus any income budgets in respect of the smaller amounts of income that units could receive). The term 'budget' was universally understood as meaning departmental **revenue expenditure budgets**. The advent of the contracting process has meant that, as well as revenue expenditure budgets being needed to reflect spending plans for staff, non-staff and capital ownership charges, **income budgets** have to be created to reflect the volume and source of anticipated contract income. If 'internal trading' is carried out between departments then **recharge budgets** are also required. This is an important development and care must be taken when discussing 'budgets' – particularly with those whose NHS career pre-dates contracting – to clarify which type or types are being referred to.

The budget setting process

Budgets normally are set on an annual basis. The purpose of the annual budget strategy is to identify, to the requisite level of detail, both the sources of income, and the expenditure plans for that income. Budgets are then set as part of an annual budget setting cycle for each of the following main headings:

- staff (both WTE and £)
- non-staff
- capital ownership costs (capital charges)
- recharges
- income.

Control of capital expenditure is equally as important as that of revenue. It is essential to plan exactly how capital funds are to be spent, not only to ensure that appropriate investment is made in buildings and equipment suitable for the intended purpose, but also because of the capital charges that will flow as a result of ownership.

The exact approach to budget setting varies locally depending on circumstances, preferences and arrangements. One possible approach is set out in the remainder of this chapter, but the aim is always the same: to provide budget managers with an appropriate level of funding for the activity, however measured, their area of responsibility is planned to undertake.

Staff budgets

Staff costs relate directly to the mix of numbers and grades of staff employed, i.e. the basic 'volume and unit cost' equation highlighted in an earlier chapter. Financial control is achieved by controlling this mix, and this process is often called **manpower control**, neatly emphasizing once again that management of finances stems only from management of resources.

There are a few more terms that need to be defined before continuing.

- **Agreed establishment** is the current maximum number of posts within a department or function against which staff appointments can be made. Normally

it is expressed in whole time equivalents (WTE), analysed by grade. Each department should have an agreed establishment for manpower control purposes.

- **Funded establishment** is the current number of posts within a department or
function, expressed in whole time equivalents (WTE) and analysed by grade, for
which funding has been provided. It is in effect the WTE budget. This differs from
the agreed establishment only if any agreed posts are unfunded.
- **Actual establishment** is the current number of posts actually occupied, expressed
in whole time equivalents (WTE) and analysed by grade. Actual establishment for
any grade should never exceed the budgeted WTE, i.e. the funded establishment,
unless there are compensating savings elsewhere and such offsetting has been
agreed.

The first task when setting a staff budget is to identify specifically how many staff
of what grade are required to provide the stated level of service. This is developed
with the budget manager and relies on the manager's experience, or the application
of recognized 'norms', or both. When reaching this decision it is important to bear in
mind that a number of staff are already in post. Whilst a budget manager may have a
certain ideal establishment, the budget setting process must reflect the fact that
the majority of staff, if not all, have permanent contracts of employment. They
cannot easily be replaced with a different mix of staff grades unless some form of
redeployment is possible.

Therefore, the budget setting process would normally expect to take as its starting
point the actual establishment, for which the total gross cost of employment for a
full year is then determined. This is known as an incremental budgeting approach.
Each occupied post is costed on either a mean of scale or an actual point of scale
basis. Vacant posts within the agreed establishment may also be included for funding,
or it may be decided to change the agreed establishment by varying the number of
vacant posts to reflect anticipated activity levels for the year.

Vacancies agreed for funding cannot, by definition, be costed on an actual point of
scale basis, and it may be agreed to fund them for a full or part year at the mean of
scale, the bottom of the scale or at the actual point of scale when an appointment is
made. A vacant post may remain unfunded where it is considered either that it
should not be filled during the year or that the approval to proceed with an
appointment should be given later, as part of the overall budget strategy finalization,
when income levels agreed with purchasers are clearer. In the latter case it is still
necessary to cost the post for inclusion in the contract pricing exercise.

Where actual point of scale costing, possibly combined with funding of vacancies,
has been applied it may be decided then to reduce the total staff budget derived by a
percentage **vacancy factor** to reflect the fact that inevitable staff turnover during
the year will result in fortuitous savings to managers. Such savings may arise due to
the time delay between an individual terminating and a replacement starting, but
even where there is no such time lag between termination and starting the likelihood
is that the new starter will be paid at a lower point on the payscale, thereby saving
money. The actual percentage amount to be applied, if applied at all, is determined
by local staff turnover levels, and often varies between staff groups.

Finally there may be other adjustments to the staff WTE and financial budget,
resulting from anticipated developments or because of the centrally imposed requirement to meet cost improvement programme (CIP) targets. Whatever the case, it is
essential that a budget manager is absolutely clear as to how the funded establishment has been determined and how the actual funding provided relates to this WTE

Pharmacy department budget 19X3/X4	Funded WTE	£
STAFF		
Principal pharmacist	1.00	35 000
Senior I pharmacist	1.00	25 000
Senior II pharmacist	3.50	63 000
Basic grade pharmacist	8.50	102 000
Senior technician	3.00	36 000
Technician	5.00	50 000
Storeman	1.00	9 000
Secretarial	1.30	12 000
		332 000
Less vacancy factor @ 2%		(6 640)
Net staff budget	24.30	325 360

Figure 9.1 A typical departmental staff budget.

budget. Without this clarity, proper manpower control and hence financial control is impossible.

A typical department's staff budget may look as set out in Figure 9.1. Each budget line should be capable of being backed up with a costing for each post within the total WTE. This emphasizes the principle that the level of detail used in undertaking the budget setting process is often at a lower level than that used for monitoring budget performance.

Presentation varies locally. In Figure 9.1, it is not immediately apparent that the previously funded establishment of 5.60 WTE technicians has been reduced by 0.60 WTE as part of the year's CIP savings. One alternative approach is specifically to identify such reductions within the budget as a separate line.

This provides an annual budget. Budget performance is monitored on a much more frequent basis – usually monthly. The annual budget therefore has to be divided into twelve monthly budgets. This is known as budget phasing or profiling, and for staff budgets the most common division is into equal twelfths.

Budgets are merely the financial expressions of resource consumption plans. When constructing a budget the concern is with identifying levels of resource consumption and identifying the cost of such consumption. Over time such costs generally tend to increase, either through pay awards or through general price inflation. It is therefore important when setting budgets to determine the price base at which they are to be set. Budgets normally are set at the out-turn level of the previous year, i.e. without any inflation for the coming year included.

For staff budgets the use of out-turn costs means reflecting the current rates of pay. As this detailed calculation part of the budget strategy tends to be undertaken well before the start of a financial year, the budgets for the 19X3/X4 financial year would be calculated using the 19X2/X3 pay rates. The 19X3/X4 budget strategy then has to include an assessment of likely pay increases for each staff group for inclusion in contract prices, but the additional costs are not normally fed into budgets until the new pay rates are paid during the year. When each award is announced the impact of that on each budget line in cost terms can be calculated, either as a percentage uplift or by recalculating the new cost of each post in the funded establishment and resetting the budgets. It is crucial that the additional wage award funding is fed into the staff budget only when the increased rate actually has started to be paid, otherwise a false financial position results. If the award is announced later in the year, staff may be due arrears. The phasing of the additional funding should reflect this.

Non-staff budgets

Although non-staff costs constitute a much lower proportion of a provider's total costs, they tend to be far more diversified in nature and, arguably, can be more difficult to control. The same basic principles apply when determining a non-staff budget as with the staff budgets. First the application of the 'volume and unit cost' equation requires an assessment to be made of the level of workload to be imposed upon the department or function in the coming year; a determination of the volume of non-staff inputs required to achieve this can then be made. When this volume of inputs is costed, it becomes the basic non-staff budget.

In reality, rather than using any form of zero-based approach, the overall assessment is likely to be based predominantly upon managerial experience and an application of incremental budgeting, with prior year expenditure figures being adjusted at the margins to reflect changes in departmental workload or activity levels between the two years.

The actual main workload factor determining such incremental changes varies between non-staff headings. For some, such as drugs, CSSD and medical and surgical supplies and equipment, it is patient volume and case mix. For other headings there is not such a direct link with patient numbers; for example, heating costs may be anticipated to rise because the size of the site has been enlarged for some purpose other than directly accommodating patients.

It is a matter of experience to determine for each budget the appropriate volume measure and the main factor determining change in resource consumption levels. This requires an understanding and knowledge of **cost-behaviour** patterns. Allowance must then be made for the following:

- any changes anticipated between years in the main factor influencing activity level
- any non-recurring items
- anticipated developments
- the effect of inflation between the two years.

This approach is summarized in Figure 9.2.

A zero-based approach tends to be used more where sophisticated case mix systems are capable of providing very detailed non-staff costing information upon which to base projected budgets. Providers with such information systems are able to build non-staff cost/activity relationships, and hence budgets, in a far more refined way.

The monthly phasing of many non-staff budgets is not in equal twelfths. For example, energy bills may be received quarterly, and they can be expected to be higher in the winter period than during the summer. The energy budget therefore

Drugs costs:	£000
Total spend in 19X2/X3	300
Less: non-recurring items in 19X2/X3	−20
Plus: full-year effect of 19X2/X3 inflation	7
Plus: new developments in 19X3/X4	40
Plus: increased patient activity between years (excluding developments)	6
Projected cost in 19X3/X4	333

Figure 9.2 Calculating non-staff costs based on prior year spend (the incremental approach).

has to be phased to match that pattern of energy consumption. In the winter months, there may be a higher incidence of chest complaints requiring certain types of antibiotics. If this is a material amount then it is worth phasing that element of the drugs budget to match the anticipated pattern of antibiotic use.

Non-staff budgets must also be calculated to reflect current price levels, that is the prices pertaining on the first day of the financial year. If the budget calculations are being undertaken before the start of the financial year then, whichever approach is being adopted, an allowance has to be made for any increases in prices between the point of calculation and the first day of the new financial year. During the financial year additional money will be added in to the non-staff budgets each month to reflect the impact of inflation. Most financial systems are capable of undertaking this calculation and budget update automatically, on the basis of percentage inflation uplifts. These percentage uplifts may be extracted from the Health Service Price Index (HSPI). This is produced monthly by the Department of Health and sets out the month on month price increases over the major non-staff subjective headings.

Even though the actual inflation for the coming year will not be known until during the year, it is still important that an estimate of both the full-year effect and the part-year effect of it is determined for the budget strategy for inclusion in contract prices. Both current year 'part year' and prior year 'all year' effects must be considered.

Capital charges budgets

Both the depreciation and interest elements of capital charges require some form of budgetary control to ensure that the level of actual charges incurred can be monitored against planned. Where a computerized asset register is being properly maintained, an accurate assessment of depreciation and interest payable for the coming year is straightforward, and the amounts so calculated can be used to determine the total capital charges budgets.

Computerized registers normally are capable of identifying assets such as equipment to physical locations allowing capital charges budgets to be derived, at least for the depreciation element of the charge, for each of the designated budget managers. Reasonably, budget managers should only be given responsibility for assets over which they have control of acquisition, use and replacement. Responsibility for the charge relating to buildings probably would not be divided across departmental budget managers but would be allocated to a single budget manager, such as the manager responsible for the works function.

The interest payable element may be managed centrally within the provider, with a single 'budget' representing the assessed level of interest payable against which can be compared actual interest paid during the year. However, there is nothing to preclude budgets being set at departmental or functional level.

The budget strategy for the financial year also has to make allowances for anticipated changes in the level of assets held during the coming year, and for the indexation that will take place in asset values to reflect their current costs. The indices used to determine this uplift are also provided regularly by the Department of Health.

Capital budgets

One of the purposes of the business planning process is to produce a **capital invest-ment programme** (often known as a capital plan). The capital programme is divided into a number of individual capital schemes, identifying their respective allocation within the overall programme, i.e. their maximum expenditure limit. Spending against schemes is monitored on an individual basis and in that sense each capital scheme's allocation is in effect the 'budget' for that scheme. Capital budgets are not normally allocated to individual functional or departmental budget managers. Instead control over capital investment is retained centrally within a trust.

A part of the total capital monies available is that relating to the redefinition of revenue expenditure from the former £7500 upper limit to the revised lower limit, currently £5000. This element of the total capital may be controlled by setting specific 'minor capital' budgets for purchase of items such as minor medical equipment.

Determining the correct monthly phasing of each capital budget is essential because it would not normally be expected that capital amounts would be spent in equal twelfths over the year. This may not be possible in advance and commonly it is subject to ongoing review throughout the year as payments are made against schemes.

Recharges budgets

The individuals responsible for the financial management of each of the many support departments necessary for the provision of patient care are nearly always different from those responsible for taking the decisions that result in resources being consumed within such departments. This mismatch can be overcome by a policy of **recharging**, sometimes known as **cross-charging**, between departments, whereby the actual cost of work undertaken by one department, service centre or directorate on behalf of another is calculated and passed on. The disadvantage of this method is that, unless the standard costing approach is applied, there tends to be little incentive for the 'supplier' to control costs because everything spent will simply be passed on to another budget.

Service level agreements are a much more sophisticated approach and can be likened to internal 'contracts' to provide a certain level or volume of service at an agreed rate. One main attraction lies in their ability to provide a means of clearly separating financial responsibility for demand for the service from that for its efficient supply.

The detailed aspects of costing and pricing service level agreements are discussed elsewhere in this book, but once the total direct cost of a function or service is determined at the planned level of activity or workload, suitably detailed staff and non-staff revenue budgets can be set. It is then also possible to calculate an average, or 'standard', cost for each unit of activity. The standard cost becomes, in effect, the 'selling price' of each unit, with receiving departments or directorates becoming 'purchasers'. The total planned sales are, by definition, equal to the total planned revenue spend and can be reflected in the supplying function's budget statements as a series of negative 'recharges out' budgets, each identifying the income due from a particular 'purchaser'.

Each 'purchaser' is provided with a positive 'recharges in' budget to reflect the cost consequences of their planned level of demand. This should be equal to the standard price per unit multiplied by the number of units planned to be purchased. Figure 9.3 provides an example.

The consultant radiologist, in discussion with medical colleagues, has determined that the volume of radiology required for 19X3/X4 to meet anticipated patient contracts will be 100 000 weighted units (where each different type of X-ray has its own weighted unit value), analysed as follows:

	Planned demand (units)
General surgery	25 000
General medicine	30 000
Child health	15 000
Gynaecology	10 000
Respiratory medicine	20 000
Total	100 000

On this basis the radiology directorate staffing and non-staffing requirement is determined and costed, and the following budget agreed:

Radiology budget statement 19X3/X4	WTE	Activity units	£ Budget
Expenditure:			
Staff	28.5		400 000
Non-staff			100 000
Capital charges			100 000
Total expenditure budget		100 000	600 000

Figure 9.3 Budgeting for recharges out.

From the data in Figure 9.3 a crude standard cost per weighted unit can be calculated as (£600 000/100 000) = £6 per unit. The constituent elements of this standard cost are:

	£
Staff costs	4.00
Non-staff (consumables)	1.00
Capital charges	1.00

The 'recharges out' budget for radiology can then be analysed by clinical directorate on the basis of their individual 'demands'. The radiology budget statement for the year is given in Figure 9.4. A budget statement for one of the clinical directors may look as Figure 9.5.

Note how the final amount shown on the radiology budget statement is nil. This does not mean that the manager has no budget and hence no budget responsibility. The important principle to appreciate is that there are a number of equal and opposite budgets, each of which must be understood, managed and controlled.

Variance analysis, discussed in the previous chapter, provides an invaluable tool for subsequent analysis of budget performance for both the 'supplying' and 'purchasing' departments. The above approach to recharge budgeting allows a clear split of responsibility for price and usage variances.

In this case the consultant radiologist is responsible for the cost of each X-ray examination and will have to account for the 'price' elements of any overall variance. A price variance could arise in a number of ways, but primarily occurs where either the volume or unit cost of resource inputs differs from the 'standard', or planned

Radiology budget statement 19X3/X4	*WTE*	*Activity units*	*£* *Budget*
Expenditure:			
Staff	28.5		400 000
Non-staff			100 000
Capital charges			100 000
Total expenditure budget		100 000	600 000
Recharges out:			
General surgery		−25 000	(150 000)
General medicine		−30 000	(180 000)
Child health		−15 000	(90 000)
Gynaecology		−10 000	(60 000)
Respiratory medicine		−20 000	(120 000)
Total recharges out		(100 000)	(600 000)
Net budget	28.5	0	0

Figure 9.4 Radiology budget analysed by clinical directorate.

General surgery budget statement 19X3/X4	WTE	Activity units	£ Budget
Expenditure:			
Staff	63.5		730 000
Non-staff			3 000
Capital charges			25 000
Total expenditure budget			758 000
Recharges in:			
Radiology		25 000	150 000
Pathology		112 000	124 000
Pharmacy		14 000	175 000
Theatres		1 000	550 000
Total recharges in		152 000	999 000
Total budget			1 757 000

Figure 9.5 Clinical directorate budget statement.

amount. For example, an unusually difficult examination may have taken far more time than would normally be expected, or staff shortages caused by sickness may have resulted in staff of a higher grade than normal undertaking an examination. The clinical directors are responsible for the number of X-ray examinations requested and hence are accountable for any usage variance, unless inefficiencies or other problems in the radiology department or elsewhere have led to exposures having to be redone.

The practical application of the 'flexible' approach to budgeting has both advantages and potential pitfalls. These are discussed in more detail later in the chapter.

Income budgets

Following production of the preliminary tariff of contract prices, the final stages of contract negotiation can commence. When such negotiation is finalized, a provider will have a clear idea as to the level of income expected, from which purchaser and for which contracts (at whatever level defined). In the same way that it is possible to set revenue budgets it is also possible, and advisory, to set income budgets to ensure that a matching between planned income and actual income takes place.

Income budgets can be set in different formats depending on local preference, but normally they will be set in such a way as to identify, as a minimum, the total amount expected from each purchaser. Where this approach is more developed there can be an individual budget report produced for each purchaser, with the income expected from each individual contract (e.g. specialty) identified on a line-by-line basis. Another approach is to produce a budget report in respect of each clinical directorate or equivalent and to identify the income expected from each purchaser on a line-by-line basis.

The local management arrangements are the major influence on the design of the income budget reports. In terms of individual income budgets, the designated budget manager varies locally and could either be, for example, the provider's business manager or this responsibility could be delegated down to the level of individual directorates or their equivalent.

Achieving and maintaining a balanced budget strategy

It has previously been stressed that budgets are plans expressed in financial terms. The process of reflecting overall service delivery plans in detailed budgets is commonly referred to as defining the **budget strategy** for the period in question. The proper planning of service delivery requires that a strategy for funding acquisition and for resource consumption be identified and agreed. Funding and expenditure plans cannot be considered in isolation from each other; a provider must balance these, thereby identifying a funding source for all expenditure. This need can thus be described as achieving a **balanced budget strategy**, and is a critical requirement of any organization.

Prior to the introduction of contracting arrangements, a unit's budget strategy would have been completed by balancing the historical allocation, as uplifted for inflation, developments, etc., to the total funding requirement set out in the first draft of its revenue budgets. Any difference between the two amounts would have been adjusted for either by increasing or by reducing budgets at the margins as felt appropriate by the unit management, in line with agreed priorities.

The major impact on this process of the contracting arrangements is that funding is no longer provided in the form of a historical allocation. It must be secured through the provision of care, either as part of agreed patient contracts or through extra contractual referrals (ECRs), with perhaps a relatively small part coming from other sources, such as income generation schemes. Achieving a balanced budget strategy now takes on a new importance, and the most fundamental requirement of the revised process is that **the total planned level of cost incurrence must be funded by an equivalent level of secured income**.

Achieving a balanced strategy

This requires contracts to be agreed that identify the planned level of activity, the total price to be charged and paid for that activity and preferably a clear agreement as to adjustments to income receivable where actual activity differs from planned activity. Internal service level agreements are identical in concept, and should be defined equally as clearly.

The preliminary contract pricing exercise conducted before finalization of contract negotiations reflects costs based on an anticipated quantity and quality of service delivery, analysed by purchasers. This exercise may also include budgets or reserves

Budget strategy for the financial year 19X4/X5			
Expenditure	*£000*	*Income*	*£000*
Clinical directorate 1:		Purchaser 1	17 200
Medical staff	350	Purchaser 2	2 250
Ward 1 (inc. recharges)	3 450	Purchaser 3	1 200
Ward 2 (inc. recharges)	3 480	Purchaser 4	800
Clinical directorate 2:		Purchaser 5	600
Medical staff	370	Purchaser 6	200
Ward 3 (inc. recharges)	4 580	Purchaser 7	150
Ward 4 (inc. recharges)	4 520	ECRs	100
Hotel services	2 300		
Management	500		
Energy	600		
Works maintenance	1 880		
Rates	350		
Planned developments (reserves):			
Bereavement counsellor	20		
Increased nursing staffing	100		
	22 500		22 500

Notes:
1. All support services such as pathology, radiology, theatres, etc., are assumed to have zero net budgets, with recharge of their costs to clinical directorates.
2. The increase in nursing staff is proposed to increase the quality of the service.
3. Anticipated levels of ECRs have to be included in the budget strategy.

Figure 9.6 Example balanced budget strategy.

for certain developments that it is hoped to agree with purchasers. Even at this point there should be a balanced strategy. A typical budget strategy, but greatly simplified for the purpose of illustration, is shown in Figure 9.6.

When contracts are finally agreed with all purchasers, the provider is then in the position of knowing actual total income and an analysis of it by purchaser. This may well differ from the original expectations: perhaps certain proposed developments are not approved or other unexpected developments are; activity requirements may be lower or higher than first discussed; a greater switch from in-patient to day-case work may be required. Whatever the case, all changes to anticipated income levels must be properly reflected, both in the income budgets and the revenue budgets. This has to be so, quite logically, because the basic principle is that contracts reflect planned and agreed service delivery and associated income, and expenditure budgets reflect the associated planned and agreed costs, and the two must balance. Thus, for example, if the contracted activity level is lower than that originally expected and costed, the total actual costs incurred will be lower, to the extent of the variable cost

Budget strategy for the financial year 19X4/X5				
Expenditure	£000	Income	£000	
Clinical directorate 1:		Purchaser 1	16 840	
Medical staff	350	Purchaser 2	2 220	
Ward 1 (inc. recharges)	3 450	Purchaser 3	1 190	
Ward 2 (inc. recharges)	3 480	Purchaser 4	800	
Clinical directorate 2:		Purchaser 5	600	
Medical staff	370	Purchaser 6	200	
Ward 3 (inc. recharges)	4 280	Purchaser 7	150	
Ward 4 (inc. recharges)	4 520	ECRs	100	
Hotel services	2 300			
Management	500			
Energy	600			
Works maintenance	1 880			
Rates	350			
Approved developments				
Bereavement counsellor	20			
	22 100		22 100	

Notes:

1. The impact of the proposed nursing staff increase included in the original strategy for each of the main purchasers was as follows:

   Purchaser 1   £60 000
   Purchaser 2   £30 000
   Purchaser 3   £10 000

2. The revised income calculations for Purchaser 1, provided as an example, are as follows:

	£000
Original expectation	17 200
Deduct: nurse staffing	(60)
reduced activity, Ward 3	(300)
Revised income expectation	16 840

Figure 9.7 Revised budget strategy.

element. Budgets based on the original costs must be reduced as appropriate to the detailed analysis of the overall variable cost reduction.

Continuing the illustration, Figure 9.7 presents the strategy set out in Figure 9.6 following completion of contract negotiations. It has been indicated by each of the main purchasers (purchasers 1–3) that the increased nurse staffing is not affordable. Only these three purchasers contract for services that are affected by this proposal. Purchaser 1 has contracted for £300 000 less in-patient activity than expected from specialties provided by Ward 3. The budget strategy has therefore to be revised to reflect the agreed position.

Following completion of all contract negotiations the final balanced budget strategy should therefore clearly set out the agreements reached, both with purchasers in terms of patient activity levels and income, and with budget managers in terms of their budgeted functional/departmental activity levels and funding.

Maintaining a balanced strategy

A balanced budget strategy must be agreed prior to the start of each financial year. That, though, is not the end of the matter. A balanced strategy must continue to exist for the entire year, being updated to reflect changing conditions and circumstances, and responses to pressures and competing demands. The budget strategy must reflect the business strategy at **all** times, not just on the first of April each year.

The maintenance of a balanced budget strategy requires that budgets are regularly and properly revised to reflect the latest planned expenditure and income levels at the requisite level of detail. Frequently changes to individual budgeted amounts will stem from transfers of funding between budget heads, termed budget 'virement'. On other occasions this may stem from movement of funds from specific or general reserves to functional budgets. These updates do not alter the total funding availability: they merely redistribute it.

Less frequently, a provider may agree to undertake additional and unplanned contract activity, such as waiting list initiatives, utilizing spare capacity. This increases total income and hence total available funding. Central guidance stipulates that the price for such additional work should be calculated on the basis of marginal, rather than full, costs. These costs are built up using one or more of the accepted costing techniques. The overall effect of this should be that total actual income and total actual expenditure levels increase by exactly the same amount. In practice it is difficult to price additional work at that level of accuracy and prove the true marginal costs one way or the other.

Changes in activity need to be reflected in both the income budgets and the expenditure budgets to prevent distorted positions being reported in either of them. This is illustrated in Figure 9.8, which uses an example continuing from the position shown in Figure 9.7.

The position that now occurs, assuming completion of the new agreement in Figure 9.8, can be presented in two ways in the budget strategy. Both of these are shown in Figure 9.9.

The main problem with following method 1 in Figure 9.9 is that it unfairly presents expenditure budgets as overspending. This can cause much dissatisfaction amongst budget managers, for obvious reasons. Method 2 is a much fairer reflection of the true state of the income and expenditure budgets. In practice, some providers may be tempted to use method 1, with all variations from original expectation being shown as variances, whatever their cause. This is because it is simpler and avoids the sometimes onerous task of distributing additional income over expenditure budgets. However, if the marginal costing exercise has been properly conducted, these marginal costs should be capable of analysis by budget, with the result that the method 2 approach should not really be that much of a difficulty.

Assume that in October 19X4 a waiting list initiative is agreed with Purchaser 2 for 100 additional general surgery cases to be treated. All general surgery patients are treated on Ward 1. The marginal cost has been calculated to be £100 000, and the additional expenditure incurred will be reflected only in the Ward 1 budget. All expenditure and income budgets have been performing exactly as expected, and all variances are nil.

To avoid lengthy repetition of detail, the budget position that would have resulted at the end of 19X4/X5 **without the new agreement** can be summarized as follows:

Summary budget strategy and position
for the financial year 19X4/X5

	Budget £000	Actual £000	Variance £000
Expenditure budgets:			
Ward 1	3 450	3 450	0
All other budget heads	18 650	18 650	0
Total	22 100	22 100	0
Income budgets:			
Purchaser 2	2 220	2 220	0
All other purchasers	19 880	19 880	0
Total	22 100	22 100	0
Overall position			0

Figure 9.8 Reflecting additional income in the budget strategy.

Budgeting for extra contractual referrals (ECRs)

The overall contract pricing exercise takes account of the anticipated, or 'planned', level of ECR activity and its consequent impact on expenditure. The 'standard' price calculated for each ECR therefore includes an element of the total anticipated fixed costs, because fixed costs should be recovered through the total planned levels of activity (i.e. both agreed contract and estimated ECR volumes).

ECRs are always charged at full cost, regardless of their volume. If actual ECRs exceed 'planned' (estimated) ECRs, then an over-recovery of fixed costs results so that a surplus is generated (and vice versa). The greater the level of additional activity, the greater the amount of this over-recovery which results. Now consider the impact of this on the budget strategy. Assuming all other things remain equal, and setting aside the practical difficulty of deciding specifically which patients represent the over-achievement:

- If the method 1 approach illustrated in Figure 9.8 is applied to any over-achievement, those budgets that include the variable costs elements of the total cost will show an overspend, i.e. demonstrate an adverse variance. This will be

Method 1: No update of original budgets

Summary budget strategy and position for the financial year 19X4/X5

	Budget £000	Actual £000	Variance £000
Expenditure budgets:			
Ward 1	3 450	3 550	100 A
All other budget heads	18 650	18 650	0
Total	22 100	22 200	100 A
Income budgets:			
Purchaser 2	2 220	2 320	100 F
All other purchasers	19 880	19 880	0
Total	22 100	22 200	100 F
Overall position			0

With this approach the additional expenditure is reflected as an adverse, or unfavourable, variance on the expenditure budgets, whilst the additional income reflects as a favourable variance on the income reports. The overall position remains balanced, because the two variances offset each other.

Method 2: Update of original budgets

Summary budget strategy and position for the financial year 19X4/X5

	Budget £000	Actual £000	Variance £000
Expenditure budgets:			
Ward 1	3 550	3 550	0
All other budget heads	18 650	18 650	0
Total	22 200	22 200	0
Income budgets:			
Purchaser 2	2 320	2 320	0
All other purchasers	19 880	19 880	0
Total	22 200	22 200	0
Overall position			0

With this approach the nil variances are retained.

Figure 9.9 Alternative revised budgets.

more than offset by the favourable variances on the income budgets. The budgets containing the fixed costs elements will remain in balance.

- If the method 2 approach is applied, and budgets are updated on the basis of the full cost, those budgets bearing the fixed costs will underspend by the amount of the over-recovery. This is a true underspend, but for those budgets a fortuitous one.

Thus neither of these two approaches is strictly correct in its application of responsibility accounting. Local variations may exist to overcome this: for example, the over-recovered fixed overheads may be retained in a reserve. Commonly, the method 1 approach prevails, especially where ECR volumes are low, simply because of the practical difficulties and effort required to apply method 2 or a variation of it.

Budgeting for inflation

There is one other important aspect involved in the finalizing and maintaining of the budget strategy. When contract prices are derived, the planned costs must include anticipated inflation for the coming year. Expenditure budgets normally are set at current cost levels. If this were not the case the true financial position in the earlier part of the year would be distorted by false underspends arising, for example, by including the anticipated cost of a wage award in a budget prior to its being announced and paid. This results, in the earlier part of the year, in an imbalance between the total income and total expenditure budgets set, the difference being the overall amount included in prices for inflation. When total contract income is finally agreed, and all budget adjustments completed, that difference will still exist. To balance both sides of the equation, the total amount included for inflation in the agreed income is placed in a special 'budget', more commonly called an **inflation reserve**. Note also the subtle but important point that any adjustments to budgets as a result of the contract negotiation process must be actioned at current, and not inflated, costs.

The funding available for inflation is then held in the reserve and fed into budgets as required for each heading. If, during the year, inflation is higher overall than expected, there will be insufficient funding in the reserve to meet the actual inflationary costs. This presents the provider with the task of funding this shortfall. If this funding cannot be found, a deficit will occur at the year-end. Conversely, a lower than expected rate of inflation will result in an unplanned surplus, which might be applied to relieve any pressures on specific budgets or on budgets in general, or may be retained as a buffer for the coming year's round of contract negotiations.

In practice the amount initially set aside for inflation may differ from that incorporated in contract prices. If a provider's board, on the advice of the director of finance, considers that inflation will be higher than the rate agreed during contract negotiations they may prudently decide to set aside a higher amount. This will require one or more budgets to be reduced so as to ensure that the budget strategy remains balanced overall.

Fixed and flexible budgeting – the advantages and pitfalls

Fixed budgets were for many years the traditional approach to NHS budgeting. These were set at the start of the year and left unchanged apart from adjustments for pay awards, inflation and any service developments. No account was taken of general changes in activity levels, and especially of patient volumes. Performance was assessed on the basis of the 'bottom line' – was the budget over- or underspent?

Despite having the advantage of being simple to implement and understand, the fixed budget approach has long been difficult to justify in the complex and interactive business of patient care delivery. The development of case-mix management systems, driven by standard costs 'charged' to patients, provided a major step forward for those with such technology, and has undoubtedly assisted the development of the concept of flexible budgeting and detailed variance analysis in the NHS. However, a fixed unit revenue allocation ultimately worked against the philosophy because no additional funding would be available actually to put into budgets. The flexing thus became notional and hence, to many non-financial staff, a meaningless paper exercise.

With funding following the patient this has changed. It is now even more important that budgets accurately reflect the planned delivery of patient care, respond to changes in those plans and reflect the real causes of financial variances if proper sense is to be made of them. Thus the flexing of budgets to reflect agreed changes in activity has a major advantage in allowing for a far more meaningful determination of management responsibility for variances. This applies both to the financial assessment of external patient care contracts and internal service level agreements. This approach, when properly implemented and combined with variance analysis, can serve as an incentive to budget managers by fairly apportioning 'blame' and 'commendation'.

There are certain pitfalls of flexible budgeting to be aware of. These centre around the fact that standard costs or prices generally are used as the basis of charging for recharges between departments and functions. These standard costs normally include a proportion of the fixed costs of the 'supplying' department. These fixed costs are only exactly 'recovered' where actual demand equates to planned or anticipated demand. If, for example, demand upon that department is lower than expected, then the 'income' it earns through its recharges will be lower than expected and its fixed costs will be under-recovered, leading to an overspend on that budget. Staff costs can be considered as 'fixed' in the shorter term, given that staff generally cannot be taken on and laid off as demand fluctuates.

Overall at this point and all other things being equal, this may not matter to the provider because there should then be an equal and opposite underspend on the 'recharges inward' budget of the 'purchasing' department. Taken together the net position is one of breakeven. An over-demand upon the supplying department results in it underspending, but there is an equal and opposite overspend on the purchasing department. The potential pitfalls lie in whether this truly reflects the position, and what may then happen to those under- and overspends. Consider the following illustrative scenarios, which are based upon the detailed calculations set out in Figures 9.4 and 9.5.

Scenario 1

Patient activity in the general surgery clinical directorate is exactly as contracted. During the year the medical staff in the directorate request 1000 fewer X-rays than planned, through better management of treatment regimes. Their 'recharges in – radiology' budget is therefore 1000 @ £6.00 = £6000 underspent at the end of the year. The radiology department receives £6000 less income than expected, but saves only the variable costs of each X-ray unit, i.e. £1.00 each – £1000 in total. Therefore the radiology budget is £5000 overspent. Overall, the provider is £1000 underspent, representing the variable costs saved as a result of fewer X-rays being taken.

If, for example, the clinical director now decides to spend the full £6000 on a piece of equipment, the provider is left with the net position of the £5000 overspend on the radiology budget.

Alternatively, if the clinical director decides that the reduction in demand can be sustained permanently, the radiology department has to spread its fixed costs in future years over fewer activity units, i.e. over 99 000 instead of 100 000. The cost per unit increases to:

	£
Staff costs	400 000
Variable costs	99 000
Capital charges	100 000
Total expenditure	599 000

Note: This assumes that radiology staffing cannot be reduced as a result of this marginal reduction in demand; in effect they become less 'efficient'.

Cost per unit in 19X4/X5 (next year) = £599 000/99 000 = £6.05

Cost to directorates in 19X4/X5 (rounded) =

		£
General surgery:	24 000 units @ £6.05 =	145 250
All others:	75 000 units @ £6.05 =	453 750
		599 000

The clinical director uses the £6000 'saving' to fund the appointment of a part-time nurse. This causes a problem because, as demonstrated, the true funding availability to the provider is £1000, and not £6000. However, in this second instance the clinical director of general surgery may still reason that the recharges for X-ray for that directorate will fall on a permanent basis from 19X4/X5 by £150 000 – £145 250 = £4750. What will not be apparent to him or her, unless properly explained, is that recharges have risen in other directorates by £453 750 – £450 000 = £3750!

Scenario 2

The converse situation could arise if demand for X-rays was higher than planned, in which case the consultant radiologist may consider that the underspend arising from the resultant over-recovery of fixed costs is available for developments. For the same reason it is not, as it is being offset by overspends, calculated at standard cost, in the clinical directorate. At best, if the increased demand relates to additional and funded contract activity such funding will be secured at marginal cost, i.e. variable cost. The provider is no better off overall. At worst, the directorate could be requesting extra X-ray examinations because of poor control over requests, or for extra patients for whom no additional funding has been secured. In such instances not even the additional variable costs being incurred are funded.

Many other scenarios could be presented, but these two simple illustrations serve to demonstrate the underlying complexities. This emphasizes the importance of educating budget managers with a proper appreciation of the basic principles of a flexible approach to budgeting, particularly one using standard costs as a basis of recharge. Otherwise, delegation of budget management without adequate controls will lead to almost certain disaster.

Conclusion

Budgets in the NHS represent costed resource consumption plans. They are essential to proper financial control and must be built upon resource consumption behaviour patterns. Budgets must be managed in the true sense of the word, not simply administered, and managers should play a prominent role in budget construction.

There are several types of budget in the NHS. The detailed approach to calculation adopted for each of these types may vary, but the basic principle is the same – the 'unit volume and cost' equation. Budgets cannot be considered in isolation; they must form part of a budget strategy, which itself reflects, the business intentions. The budget strategy is an ongoing process, being continually updated to reflect the changing environment.

Flexible budgeting and variance analysis are key management tools that assist in the proper interpretation of financial performance. Like all tools they can be misused by untrained or unskilled hands.

Questions

1. What is the fundamental resource planning rule? Why is its application so important, and in what practical ways is it applied and achieved?
2. Describe the major types of budget used in the NHS. Discuss the importance of each with particular reference to income budgets.
3. Illustrate the methodology applied in setting a staff budget.
4. Flexible budgeting has both its advantages and its potential pitfalls. Discuss and illustrate these.
*5. The costs of running the pathology department of the Midgate Trust in 19X5/X6 were as follows:

	£000
Direct costs:	
Staff costs	300
Consumables	100
Overheads and recharges inward:	
Capital charges	100
Energy	5
Housekeeping	30
Works maintenance	50
Management	15
Total costs	600

During the year the following tests were provided, measured in work units:

	Units 000
General surgery	80
Thoracic surgery	50
General medicine	60
Acute care of the elderly	30
Child health	45
Gynaecology	35
	300

The 19X5/X6 budget for the thoracic surgery directorate was as follows:

	£000
Direct costs	700
Overheads, etc.	150
Path. tests from outside laboratories	50
	900

Patient contracts remain unchanged for 19X6/X7 and it is anticipated that exactly the same volume and mix of pathology tests will be required. Assume inflation is zero.

It is decided that the costs of the pathology department will be recharged for 19X6/X7, using the standard cost as the price per unit. Flexible budgeting is in operation.

Required:
(a) Calculate the standard cost per test, analysing it between staff, consumables and overheads/recharges. Set out the budget for the pathology department and the thoracic surgery directorate for 19X6/X7.
(b) In the first week in April 19X6, after the budgets have been set and agreed, the clinical director (CD) of thoracic surgery discovers that a pathology test with a value of 20 units can be purchased from a local private laboratory for £30.00. This external price appears to be much cheaper than the internal price of £40.00 paid for the same test. In 19X5/X6 the directorate requested

1500 of these tests. The CD therefore arranges for all such tests to be purchased from the private laboratory, with the declared intention that 'the savings of £15 000 can be used toward funding a new full-time nursing post'. Assuming all other things are as planned, calculate the true impact on the finances of the trust.

10

Pricing and the internal market

AIMS

This chapter considers the application of pricing theory to the practice of the internal market in the NHS. Specifically it aims to:

- examine the concept of pricing as part of the marketing mix and how it is closely associated with costing and budgeting;
- consider the factors that influence the pricing decision, in particular the workings of the laws of supply and demand in different market conditions;
- analyse the concept of breakeven from the perspective of an NHS provider under different types of contract;
- present the limitations of economic and accounting theory in the internal market;
- contrast target pricing in commercial practice and in the NHS and outline the problem of cost-spiralling;
- examine marginal cost pricing and the need for flexibility in reaching pricing decisions.

Costing, budgeting and pricing

The term 'price' is another of those apparently familiar, everyday terms that can suddenly take on a range of meanings when discussed in detail. Perhaps the biggest confusion tends to be over the difference in meaning between 'cost' and 'price'. Consider the following definition:

> A price is the monetary value asked or paid for a specified activity or service.

There is no reference to the word 'cost' in the definition. In the commercial world the price does not have to equal the cost. The price charged is determined by what are termed **market forces**. Any difference between cost and price would be a 'profit' or a 'loss'.

Pricing in the NHS is the process by which costs are converted into prices asked or charged for patient contracts to secure income. However, when it comes to the matter of pricing patient contracts the central guidance produced by the DoH is very clear. There must be compliance with three basic principles:

- the price charged generally should equal the actual or anticipated revenue cost;
- costs should include depreciation, calculated on a straight line, current cost basis, and an interest charge of 6% on capital assets employed;
- there should be no planned cross-subsidization of cost between contracts or purchasers.

The contract pricing methodology employed must also be capable of audit, which in turn implies adequate and appropriate documentation of the process being maintained.

The first of these principles means that there should be no planned over-inflating of prices to recover in excess of cost with the intention of making a surplus, although it is accepted that an unplanned surplus (or deficit) may well arise. This is the **price equals cost** rule, which can be expressed as follows:

Total price = Total cost

A similar rule was highlighted in an earlier chapter, whereby the planned cost has to be represented by equivalent budgets. Combining these two rules produces the important principle, summarized in Figure 10.1.

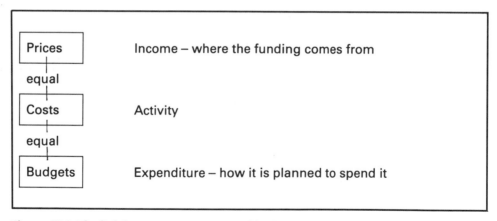

Figure 10.1 The link between prices, costs and budgets.

Budgets are used to control costs. The total budget must be set at a level within the total income generated by that level of activity. The problem facing the provider is what price to charge for each of the services it offers. In reaching this decision cost information has a key role to play, but so does other types of information available within the organization. The role of costing is to provide information on which pricing decisions can be based. However, the NHS principle of basing price primarily on cost is fundamentally different from the principles usually applied in commercial practice.

In a pure market model, price is one component of what is termed the **marketing**

mix. The customer does not buy the product if it does not meet the perceived need, or if the customer has not heard about it or cannot obtain it conveniently. So price is one of four Ps — price, product, promotion and place. Neglecting any one of these areas will impact upon the total sales income gained by the private sector firm. To what extent does this theory apply in the case of the NHS?

To answer this question it is necessary to identify the 'customer'. Ultimately this is the patient, yet normally it is the general practitioner who will decide where it is best that a patient be referred for examination or care. The GP, acting on behalf of patients, can thus better be thought of as the customer in terms of the theory. How is the GP influenced by the four Ps?

- The quality standard should be assured in the contract specification with the GP, if a fundholder, or with the DHA. If the **product** is not right then the customer will refuse to buy at any price.
- **Promotion,** as in the narrower sense of advertising the 'product availability', of the NHS is not really required, because a general public awareness already exists and more specific knowledge can easily be gained through the general practitioner. This is not to say that individual providers should not promote, or 'market', themselves in the sense of enhancing awareness of the specific services they can provide, but this is a straightforward exercise when compared to the commercial world. The providers can adopt a strategy of market segmentation where the market is divided into groups of customers which have similar attributes, such as GP fundholders. This small sub-group can be targeted in any marketing initiative and their needs established by market research.
- The **place** at which the product can be obtained is inevitably fixed by the geographical location of the hospital, health centre, etc., although there is scope for mobile provision of some treatments, and provision at home for many community services. For the patient, the place is probably the most important component, but for the purchaser, the price will be more important.

In contrast to the commercial market-place, price is of far greater relative importance in the NHS and should play a major role in determining the level of custom attracted. In practice, however, the true customers, i.e. patients, will not be the slightest bit interested in the comparative prices of different providers and may prefer treatment at one location over another for all sorts of other reasons. This can cause problems if contracts have not been negotiated with this provider, possibly because of relatively high prices. It is here that GP fundholders in particular will be faced with dilemmas.

Factors that influence the pricing decision

It would be beneficial at this point to discuss some private sector principles relating to pricing decisions as it will provide a further insight into the complexities of the NHS 'market'.

Some private firms, especially smaller businesses, will have little choice other than to accept the price indicated by similar products in the market-place. Economists state that these firms are 'price takers' and are operating in a state of **perfect competition**. The opposite end of the spectrum is the **monopoly** supplier who has total control over price and hence profit. In practice these states represent the ends

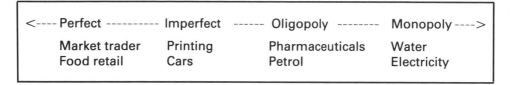

Figure 10.2 The competition continuum.

of a continuum and most firms operate in states of **imperfect competition**; in some industries, where barriers to entry are high, only a few large firms exist and this is known as an **oligopoly**. Figure 10.2 illustrates the competition continuum.

Even if the firm is a price taker then an analysis of costs is still necessary if the firm is to operate profitably. In imperfect and oligopolistic markets, non-price competition is more evident which also impacts on costs. For example, the goods 'given away' with petrol vouchers are variable costs and the advertising campaign that accompanies the offer will be a fixed cost.

Economic theory dictates that resources are allocated most efficiently in a market of perfect competition. Generally, the NHS 'internal' health care market operates under conditions of imperfect, rather than perfect, competition. Frequently, providers may find themselves in a local monopoly or local oligopoly situation where, due to scarcity of supply, what are termed 'super-profits' could be earned. Given that the market size is totally dictated by public money, cash limited by the government, benefiting from such a monopoly position in that way is unacceptable as it will lead to a less than efficient allocation of resources. This potential inefficiency is checked by the centrally imposed regulations in pricing decisions.

The intentions of the NHS contracting arrangements are to increase efficient resource allocation. This can only be fully realized if providers and purchasers act as if the market were one of perfect competition. This explains why NHS providers are required to base price so as to recover costs, which only pertains in perfect market conditions. The 'internal' market is therefore constrained to perfect competition pricing conditions even though the natural market would not allow this.

Cost/income relationships and pricing

Chapter 6 presented in graphical format the total cost curve for fixed, semi-fixed, stepped and variable costs. These serve to demonstrate the behaviour of such costs at different activity levels. One further way of using the total cost curve is to combine it with the income function to determine the output level required to cover costs incurred. This can assist in pricing decisions.

In the pre-contracting NHS the income curve was a straight line equal to the cash limit allocated to an individual unit, and expenditure generally was equal to income in that units aimed to spend all the available funds. This is shown in Figure 10.3, in which EE^1 is the total cost line and II^1 is the line representing total income. Where the lines intersect at B, the 'breakeven' level of activity, X, is reached. At activity levels higher than X, expenditure exceeded income and, as no more cash was forthcoming under this system, this increased activity would result in 'overspending' situations. This would have to be recouped from the following year's cash allocation.

At levels below X, income exceeded expenditure and 'underspends' resulted. Any cash not taken up would be 'lost', and would not be automatically made available for the next accounting period. Therefore the incentive was for managers to spend up to their cash limit and no more, with underspends regarded as much an evil as overspends.

Notice that, if the fixed costs increase, the total cost curve moves upwards parallel to the existing line. This means that the unit can only support a lower level of activity, i.e. it becomes inefficient. The opposite is true of fixed cost reductions. A hospital closure would result in fixed cost reductions and, if the patients can be treated in spare beds in another hospital, the overall level of activity can remain unaltered.

The effect of increased variable costs is an increase in the slope of the total cost line which has the same consequences as increases in fixed costs. However, there is generally more opportunity to control the variable costs at the patient level. For example, branded drugs normally are more expensive than their generic alternatives.

Under the contracting arrangements, providers derive funds by performing services for health care purchasers. There are three types of contract, the first of which, 'block', is not related to volume, while the other two, 'cost and volume' and 'cost per case', have variable elements. The same concept of breakeven still applies, but overspends will result in deficits on the income and expenditure account while underspends will result in surpluses.

- The old cash limit system is mirrored in the new **block contract**, which is a fixed sum for a defined service but not volume. The graph for this income function, Figure 10.4, is identical in shape to the line II[1] in Figure 10.3. However, there are two other types of contract which have different implications.
- **Cost per case** contracts do not have a fixed element and result in a set fee for a specific item of service. There is no commitment to meet a given level of activity. This is akin to a full market environment and produces an income curve which is not horizontal, but projects from the origin at an angle which relates to the cost per case. Figure 10.5 illustrates the intersection of the total cost curve and income curve based solely on cost per case contracts. It is at this point that cost and price are equal.
- The final type of contract is **cost and volume** which specifies the volume of service to be provided in return for a given payment and allows for additional

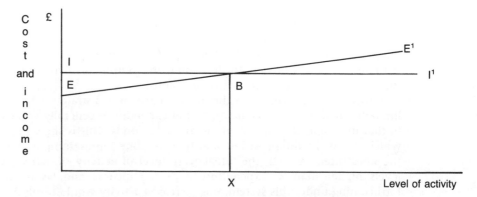

Figure 10.3 Breakeven activity level in cash limited conditions.

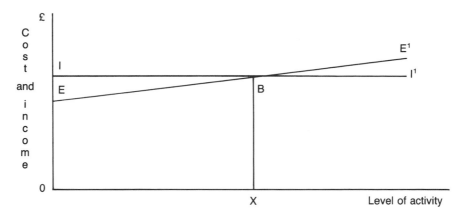

Figure 10.4 Breakeven activity level for block contracts.

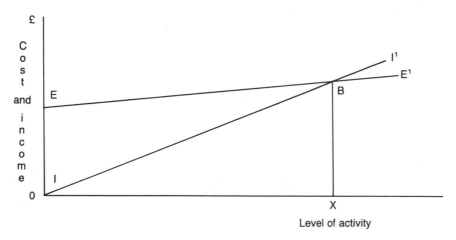

Figure 10.5 Breakeven activity level for cost per case contracts.

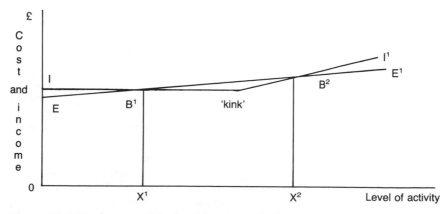

Figure 10.6 Breakeven activity level for cost and volume contracts.

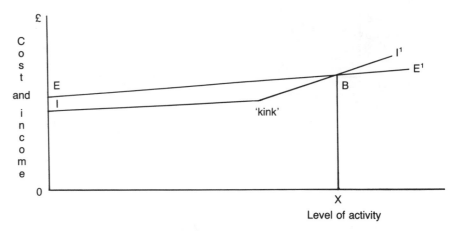

Figure 10.7 Breakeven activity level for cost and income.

payments to be made if that volume is exceeded, up to an agreed ceiling level. The income curve is therefore 'kinked' with a horizontal element followed by an upward sloping element. The 'kink' occurs at the 'base level' point specified in the cost and volume contract above which additional sums are forthcoming from the purchaser. Figure 10.6 indicates this scenario.

This kinked income function can result in two breakeven points, one occurring on the specified volume of service and one occurring when additional payments are forthcoming. Levels of activity between X^1 and X^2 are points where expenditure exceeds income, i.e. deficit situations. This places a strong emphasis on the careful management of cost and volume contracts which need to be carefully planned and monitored.

The three types of contract can be aggregated in the same way as were the different cost elements above. The bulk of the total income received will be fixed, but there will be minor variable elements and a slight 'kink' in the line. So a slightly upward sloping line is produced, as shown in Figure 10.7.

The point marked B is the breakeven point which takes account of all costs and incomes. It is located just above the 'kink' in this case, indicating that the provider must compete and win cost and volume and cost per case contracts if it is at least to break even.

Any point from the origin to point X is a level of activity which results in a deficit, i.e. the total cost exceeds total income. Any point above X results in a surplus, i.e. total income exceeds total costs. The net income earned below point X is described as 'contributing' to covering fixed costs and any point above X is contributing' to the surplus.

The high fixed elements of both cost and income means that managers must pay close attention to the control of fixed costs so that they fall within the relatively fixed income earned. Fixed costs can account for 70–80% of total cost. This is very similar to the pre-1991 cash limit scenario, only there is a contractual relationship between purchaser and provider which means that a competitive situation exists.

The relevant range and the assumption of linearity

Modelling is a simplification of the real world which can enable decisions to be made and tested in a simulated environment. The more precise the simulation then the more difficult it is to develop and the more costly to model. When developing the model, the required level of precision must be borne in mind. It is unlikely to be worthwhile modelling the costs of a hospital down to activity levels so low that they will not result in practice, nor to such high activity levels that a dramatic increase in the provider's market share and asset base would be required. For this reason, the scope of the model is restricted to the **relevant range**, which is that within which decisions are contained.

Economic theory postulates that the cost and income functions facing any organization will not be straight lines, but curved:

- **Income**. Economists argue that to increase turnover, in stable demand conditions, then price must fall. This would be the case for any DMU or trust because purchasers will buy more treatments as long as there is unsatisfied demand in the form of waiting lists. However, the total turnover is fixed nationally by a cash limit.
- **Costs**. Economists point to the law of diminishing returns as well as to concepts of economies and diseconomies of scale to argue that average cost per unit will rise above a certain point. Again, this phenomenon will apply to NHS organizations.

While the economist's theory of the firm can be looked upon as an ideal, its use in modelling would require excessive detail and, in any case, is not likely to be accurate. In practice, decisions must be reached and linearity assumptions give an adequate approximation to real life. Figure 10.8 shows the economist's cost and income functions and the linear functions of the accountant. Over the relevant range

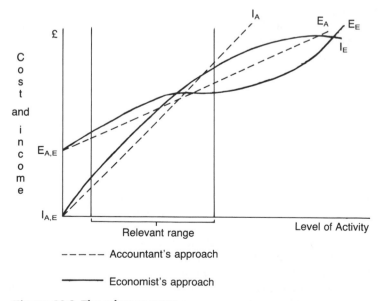

Figure 10.8 The relevant range.

the difference is small and the activity level at which breakeven is reached is very similar. However, the accountant's model is easier to construct and understand.

Limitations of the economist's pricing model

The linearity assumption for the total income function is strongly contested by economists who argue that demand is **elastic**. As the term implies, the theory of elasticity of demand hypothesizes that the quantity demanded by the market is dependent upon the price charged. Specifically it states that the lower the price charged, the higher will be the quantity demanded. In perfect market conditions this will be immediately observed as purchasers take advantage of the better price. This results in a downward sloping demand curve as shown in Figure 10.9.

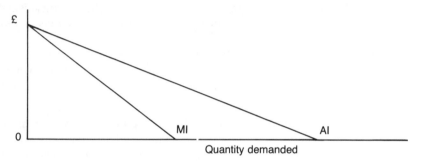

Figure 10.9 The economist's demand curve.

Sensitivity to price changes, or demand elasticity, is given by the slope of the demand curve. An inelastic demand curve would be vertical while an elastic demand curve would be horizontal. Downward sloping demand curves have elasticities that vary along their length.

Unlike the total cost function the demand curve has a negative slope. The demand curve is **not** the total income curve, but the **average income** (AI) curve. AI is defined as the total income divided by quantity. The price charged at any particular point along the curve varies and hence the **marginal income** (MI) from moving from one price to another will fall. The relationship is such that MI falls twice as fast as AI.

Given the market conditions in the NHS, where waiting lists are indicative of unsatisfied demand, there is nothing to indicate that the demand curve for patient treatment will be anything other than downward sloping. If treatment price falls then more patients will, in theory, be attracted, via their purchaser, to treatment by that provider.

However, in practice the purchaser may decide to use the funds released by price reductions to purchase different treatments. This phenomenon is termed the **income and substitution effect** by economists.

In the NHS, price changes only occur when contracts are renegotiated. Generally, prices will rise with inflation, but price reductions may occur on individual contracts if overhead apportionment bases are altered or costs savings are realized. As a consequence the regulated market will work more slowly than in conditions of perfect competition. This demonstrates that despite the regulatory mechanisms in place, the internal market remains imperfect.

Cost-based pricing

As with costing techniques, there are a variety of established pricing methodologies in the private sector. The NHS pricing mechanism is to some extent dictated by the fundamental requirement to ensure a direct relationship with cost, i.e. pricing must be 'cost-based'. A consideration of the theory and practical application both in the private sector and NHS of cost-based pricing techniques will be appropriate at this point.

The logic of **cost plus pricing** is very straightforward. The full cost of the service is identified and to it is added a percentage which represents the desired rate of return. This has given rise to the term **target pricing**. An example of a cost-based price calculation is given is Figure 10.10. On the face of it, the simplicity and apparent accuracy of cost-based pricing methods is attractive, but the main disadvantage in the private sector is the absence of any market considerations.

The approach does have a parallel in the pricing of NHS contracts in that present regulations require the price charged to equal cost (including depreciation) plus a nationally determined mark-up that recovers a return on capital investment, currently 6%. It is important to note that this is not the same as a 6% mark-up on cost. Figure 10.11 re-presents Figure 10.10 as relating to the NHS.

Another disadvantage is the allocation of overheads. To comply with the pricing

---

Total overheads or fixed costs amount to £7 500 000 and the manufacturer expects to sell 10 000 units. To recover these fixed costs the manufacturer must allocate them at (7 500 000/ 10 000 =) £750 per unit. Variable costs per unit amount to £250. The capital employed in producing these units is £20 000 000.

Cost per unit	£
Variable costs	250
Fixed costs	750
Total cost per unit	1000
Target mark-up (50%)	500
Selling price	1500

Figure 10.10 Cost-based pricing – a private sector application.

Total overheads or fixed costs amount to
£7 500 000 and the provider expects to treat 10 000
patients. To recover these fixed costs the provider
must allocate them at (7 500 000/10 000 =) £750
per patient. Variable costs per patient amount to
£250. The capital employed in delivering this
activity is £20 000 000.

Cost per patient	£
Variable costs	250
Fixed costs	750
Total cost per patient	1000
Target mark-up (6% × £20 000 000/10 000)	120
Contract price	1120

Figure 10.11 Cost-based pricing – an NHS application.

principles, providers commonly apply **full absorption** costing techniques when
pricing contracts. These techniques involve identifying total costs against total planned
activity, which should include an estimate of likely ECR levels. This identification, in
turn, requires overhead costs to be shared, or absorbed, over that planned level of
activity. Full recovery of fixed overheads is achieved only where the provider treats
exactly the number of patients it planned for.

If the provider does not estimate this number correctly then the margin for error is
high. In the example, fixed overheads accounted for 75% of total cost on which
price is based. These overheads are incurred regardless of activity levels and it is
dangerous to treat them on a cost-per-case basis. If activity levels exceed the initial
estimate then the total overheads will be **over-absorbed** because each patient
treated at the full contract price will continue to 'recover' £750 towards meeting the
fixed overheads costs, which will already have been fully recovered from achievement of the planned activity. Surpluses will therefore be generated.

Assume that 11 000 cases were treated at average cost then the total fixed costs
recovered would be £750 × 11 000 = £8 250 000, which would produce a surplus of
£750 000. The converse is also true. Assume only 9000 cases were treated then the

			Cases treated	
		9 000	10 000	11 000
Fixed costs	£	7 500 000	7 500 000	7 500 000
Fixed costs recovered	£	6 750 000	7 500 000	8 250 000
Over/(under)-recovery	£	(750 000)	–	750 000

Figure 10.12 Under- and over-recovery of overheads.

total fixed costs recovered would only be £750 × 9000 = £6 750 000, a deficit of £750 000. This relationship is shown in Figure 10.12.

Variations from planned activity chargeable at average price will most likely arise in the case of extra contractual referrals and cost-per-case contracts, because any activity above cost and volume contract levels will normally be negotiated at marginal cost.

Predicting accuracy in activity levels may be problematical. Given the fact that there are waiting lists for many treatments, under-recovery does not appear to be a problem. However, the total activity of the NHS is cash limited, unlike the private sector which faces market conditions. The real problem facing individual providers is the action of competitors who may attract patients from the existing market share, thereby causing actual activity to fall below planned.

Another major problem will probably be on the estimation and control of the allocated cost proportion. If total fixed costs are 5% higher than anticipated then fixed costs will be under-recovered by £375 000 even if actual activity is as planned. However, over-estimation of fixed costs produces an over-recovery which can be used to reduce allocation rates in future years. This will have the effect of reducing the cost per case.

There can be a vicious circle when using full absorption cost-based pricing if it results in too high a price being charged initially. The price may be so high that purchasers respond by cutting their contract activity requirements to balance to their available funding for that type of treatment. When this reduced activity level is fed back into the model the fixed costs per patient are increased, thereby pushing up the contract price. This price increase may reduce volume even further and so the problem repeats itself. This is known as **cost spiralling** and presents perhaps the greatest danger to providers in the internal market. A downward spiral can only be halted by cutting fixed costs such that total costs can be balanced to income. Any upward spiral will be halted in the short to medium term when maximum capacity is reached.

In the private sector there is also a problem with a firm that produces many products when overheads are to be apportioned amongst them. An incorrect apportionment can result in sub-optimal pricing decisions. A similar problem exists in the NHS where groups of procedures – or diagnosis related groups (DRG) – can be used as proxy 'products'. These 'products' can be aggregated in the hospital sector according to medical and surgical specialties. Community providers will have programmes of care which are conceptually similar as far as this element of the methodology applies. The specialties represent the private sector equivalent of departmental cost centres. Fixed costs are allocated to specialties using workload measurements and, given the numerous functional components of that which makes up this fixed cost, the possibilities for over- and under-recoveries are multiplied greatly.

In practice, NHS specialty costs have tended to vary enormously on an average cost-per-case basis. So much calculation is required that it is only the massive reduction in information processing costs that make any sort of costing system for the NHS a possibility at all. Commentators have pointed out that it is not just the computer hardware and software that is required, but also adequately trained staff in sufficient numbers, and this unfortunately has not been the case in most providers.

Once specialty costs have been established, further disaggregation and apportionment is necessary to incorporate the fixed costs in prices at DRG, procedure or patient level. This further widens the scope for a mismatch between fixed overhead apportionment and recovery.

Marginal cost-plus pricing

To avoid the problems of overhead allocation, some firms in the private sector use a cost-based price model that ignores fixed costs and adds a mark-up to **marginal costs**. This is sometimes referred to as **relevant cost plus pricing**. This is very common in the retail trade where the marginal costs are easily determined. The mark-up varies with the goods sold. High turnover products tend to have lower mark-ups than low turnover goods. So a grocer may apply a mark-up of 33% to the cost paid for fruit and vegetables, while a jeweller may apply over 100% to stock purchases.

Other uses of this method are in cases of short-term decision-making where full cost pricing may have been used, but now the firm needs to reduce stock levels to generate cash flow.

The method ties in very well with breakeven analysis, which is used extensively in the private sector. There is very little difference between the private sector method and the NHS prescribed method of marginal costing. The difference is that no mark-up is applied, so in theory it will not be financially beneficial for a provider to take on any contracts on a **marginal cost** basis.

As is often the case in practice, there isn't one single correct answer to the question – what is the best price? The 'best' method may not be the one that arrives at a price that maximizes surpluses, or maximizes patients treated. However, if managers are aware of the marginal cost in the short and long terms as well as full cost then they can make decisions in the light of that information. For example, waiting list initiatives undertaken during a financial year can be priced to recover marginal costs, but this is not the best method to arrive at prices for main contracts.

Pricing policy

It is through the manipulation of costing allocation and apportionments that providers will be able to influence price. If it is desired to price cheaply, this can be accomplished by underestimating costs and/or over-stating volume and under-recovering overheads. Under-pricing in this way is known as **penetration pricing** in the private sector. It is used to defeat competitors and allow for market exploitation in later accounting periods when the absence of competition permits inflated prices to be charged. This is, of course, outlawed in the NHS and cost information on which prices are based will have to be audited. By the time these controls are effective the desired result may have been achieved and such skulduggery can be expected where competition is tight.

The opposite strategy may be chosen whereby the treatments are deliberately priced at a premium, i.e. through overestimation of costs and/or underestimating volume. This may exploit the monopoly position of novel treatments. This is known as **price skimming**. In later stages, when increased competition enters the 'market', the price is lowered to reach a wider market base.

This is the sort of strategy followed in the private sector by products such as CD players or the latest advance in computers. It has the advantage of recovering quickly the overheads incurred in developing the new product and bringing it to market. It also allows cash to be generated which can be invested in production methods which may reduce manufacturing costs and allow adequate returns to made on the product when it is in the maturity and saturation phases. This cash could also be used for research and development for the next leap forward.

The parallels in the NHS are easy to find where new treatments and diagnoses abound. Once again, this is not permitted but will be difficult to prove, and given the variety of costing methods available compliance with regulations can be satisfied.

Conclusion

The determination of price in the NHS is subject to regulation due to market imperfections. The rule is broadly stated that price will equal cost and cost, by and large, will mean full cost. This constraint will result in an attempt to increase volume to reduce prices. There will be a parallel drive to reduce overheads. The increased volume and lower overheads will lead to a lower price per case. The theory, and the government's objective, is that this will result in efficiencies on the part of the provider and more patients will be treated for the same money. After all, the government determines the **size** of the market each year by means of the cash limit. However, there are behavioural implications and technical problems which have not yet been overcome. This will lead to sub-optimal aspects to the operation of the costing and budgeting system in the short term, and maybe even in the long term.

Having explored some of the theory, the next chapter places pricing in a more practical context using the theoretical underpinning developed above.

Questions

1. 'If price is market driven in the commercial world, why does the government wish to base price on costs in the NHS? Surely this is inefficient?' Discuss.
2. 'For the NHS patient, pricing treatments is irrelevant as no money changes hands. It is just a bureaucratic exercise that will lead to more administrative costs which means that less patients will be treated in the long run.' How can the cost of the pricing process be justified in commercial terms?
3. The internal market relies on the existence of waiting lists in order to work effectively. If the waiting lists disappeared then the market would collapse. Do you think the internal market will disintegrate if it is too successful?
4. 'The internal market and the idea of pricing treatments is fine in theory, but the practical realities are such that there is very little difference to the cash limit system that used to operate adequately.' Has the theory behind the internal market been manipulated too much to be of any economic relevance?
5. 'There are so many different approaches to price determination that the providers can still charge any price they like which defeats the objective of market regulation.' Discuss.

11

The pricing process in practice

AIMS

The previous chapter examined pricing theory and its applicability to the NHS internal market. This chapter provides an overview of the pricing process in practice. In particular it aims to:

- outline the two main approaches to contract costing and pricing;
- describe the stages in the pricing process;
- identify the key variables, and highlight the impact of changes in them;
- emphasize the main factors influencing price;
- consider the future of pricing by DRG.

Approaches to the costing and pricing process

Prior to the start of each financial year, as part of the budget strategy, a major contract pricing exercise has to be completed. Its aim is to identify:

- the specific 'types' of 'activity' to be undertaken
- the planned volume of that activity – this is the 'output' (or, more correctly, the 'throughput') measure
- the associated total cost – the 'input' measure.

Depending on the form of contract, this then allows a cost per unit of activity to be derived, using the simple **unit cost and volume** equation.

The specific activities contracted for are determined by the specialties, procedures and interventions that the provider is currently providing and is in a position to develop. There is a core of general activity, for which all main purchasers have a demand, with more specialist treatments at the periphery. Volumes are agreed by the contract negotiation process, and providers have a reasonable idea of total demand from each purchaser's procurement plans.

The 'unit of activity', or 'currency' as it is often referred to, is generally agreed locally for each contract type. There is no central prescription of the currency on which individual contract agreements have to be based. Certain contract monitoring returns do have to be produced and submitted to the centre on a regular basis, but this does not mean that the same currency actually has to be used for contracting. However, if it is not, then the provider has the task of maintaining records of activity in two currencies, for example deaths and discharges and finished consultant episodes. The selection of the currency is influenced by a number of factors which are discussed below.

In practice, individual providers have total freedom to agree with purchasers the main elements of the **product definition**. These elements include matters such as achievement of Patient Charter and other quality issues, as well as defining the measurement currency. This has one obvious implication, namely that price comparisons between providers can only be meaningful if the currency and the full product definition are known.

The main approaches to pricing

There are two main ways of undertaking costing for pricing purposes. These can be described as the 'bottom-up' and 'top-down' approaches.

The bottom-up approach

As the name suggests, this method starts by defining the total treatment regime for each type of output. This is then divided into its constituent parts or steps at the lowest practical level of resource consumption, e.g. time in theatre, type and quantity of drugs, pathology tests and X-ray examinations, minutes of nursing care, etc. For each of these components a standard (average) level of resource consumption is identified and costed, using input costs wherever possible. In some instances actual, rather than standard, costs may be used. Adding these costs together provides the total cost, which can be used to derive the price.

The disadvantage of this method lies in the high level of importance placed upon the need for accuracy in each of the three facets of:

- definition of treatment profiles
- measurement of resource consumption
- conversion of this into costs.

When properly and accurately applied the results should have a high level of acceptance by all those involved in the process. However, this approach relies heavily on sophisticated clinical, workload measurement and costing systems at departmental level. Its use for main contract costing and pricing is not a practical proposition for most providers, simply because either they do not have such expensive systems or, if they do, they require further development. Its main potential for use is in the area of pricing low-volume and/or high-cost, i.e. resource-intensive, interventions. Useful lessons can be learned in such instances, allowing a wider application of this approach in the future, particularly as case-mix systems develop.

The top-down approach

This method starts at the other end. It takes the highest practical level of planned or actual cost aggregations and divides these over associated output volumes, either by direct allocation or by apportionment. It provides certain advantages over the bottom-up approach:

- it is much simpler, and hence quicker and cheaper, to apply;
- the resultant prices can be directly reconciled to planned and actual costs, both by contract and in total, allowing them to be proven for audit purposes.

It is likely to be less accurate than bottom-up costing, and can lead to credibility problems with clinical staff in particular if they feel that the resultant prices bear no relation to their perception of costs. Despite this, its use is widespread, but primarily because of the lack of a viable alternative rather than its advantage of simplicity.

The remainder of this chapter examines the pricing process based primarily upon the top-down approach. As with other topics, it is the principles involved rather than the specific details of the process being described that are of importance. These apply equally whichever approach is used in practice.

Stages in the pricing process

The budget strategy requires an identification of all costs to a sufficient degree of analysis to allow the setting of budgets. It is then possible to take each of these, in part or in whole, and to allocate and apportion them all to contract activity using the basic costing principles. Budgets are, after all, simply planned costs. Not only does this make the task less arduous and repetitive, but ensures that no costs are over-looked. All costs must be so matched against patient activity, otherwise the total prices charged will not equal total costs.

The difficulty of this task will depend upon the level at which contracts are struck. So, before starting the pricing exercise, the first decision to resolve is, at which level should contracts be struck?

At which level should contracts be struck?

A basic principle is that contracts should not be struck at a level below which meaningful prices can be produced. For providers with many disparate clinical specialties or types of clinical service a single, common price per patient for all specialties/services would be a very poor basis on which to contract. At the very least some account has to be taken of the specialty and intervention type (in-patient, out-patient, day case, etc.), and prices have to be produced for the GP fundholder chargeable procedures. However, this simple approach which, for example, gives a single price for, say, all patients seen in a particular specialty leaves two questions unresolved:

- Should prices be derived at lower levels, such as sub-specialties, diagnosis related groups (DRGs), or individual procedures?

- Should a more sensitive form of analysis be used at the specialty level – for example, using a number of relative severity bandings within each specialty?

There are no correct answers to these question and the decision as to the level at which contracts should be priced is influenced by a number of local considerations. Their resolution is, however, governed by two limiting factors:

- The first factor is the ability to obtain suitable and accurate functional activity/ workload information at the various levels at which it may be desired to derive prices, so as to allow the allocation and apportionment of costs or budgets. For example, assume the pharmacy department is able to produce accurate historic drug cost data by specialty at ward level but cannot further analyse it by the patient groupings for which it is hoped to contract. There is thus no sound basis for deriving anticipated drugs costs for inclusion within contract prices at that lower level. Unless a huge manual exercise is undertaken, some form of apportionment based upon various judgements has to be used and, depending upon the materiality of the amount both in absolute and relative terms, this may invalidate the exercise. There are many costs which would require this level of analysis and without adequate computerization the task soon becomes hopeless.
- The second factor is again linked to the capability of systems: this time the capability of the provider's operational activity recording system to identify each patient to a contract such that actual performance against contract can be measured. There is little point agreeing contracts at procedure level or using a severity banding system within a specialty if the mechanism by which individual patients are matched to a contract cannot, or does not, correctly provide that degree of analysis. A provider may be able to produce the most accurate and refined contract prices for every possible test, procedure, treatment and intervention, but this is of little benefit to the contracting process if the operational system for recording contract activity is not equally accurate and refined. This may be because inadequately trained or inappropriate staff have the responsibility of matching patients to contracts, or because the technology is under-developed. Whatever the case, there are few things more frustrating to those involved with the contracting process than when the contract performance figures clearly lack credence and cannot be relied upon. In the contracting environment activity recording techniques are every bit as important as pricing methodologies and the two must be developed in parallel.

Cost analysis

Once the level of cost analysis has been decided, the pricing process is broken down into a number of stages, the actual number depending upon the decision. The first stage is to analyse all costs, as represented in budgets, to specialty or directorate level, or the local equivalent.

A large part of a provider's costs is either reflected in, or is capable of easy allocation to, directorate or specialty type budgets, particularly if internal service level agreements or cruder inter-departmental cross-charging arrangements are in place. Where this is not the case some costs/budgets associated with one functional department may have to be apportioned to directorates via another function, because not all of their activity will be in direct support of directorates or specialties.

Table 11.1 Analysis of provider's total budgets by directorate (financial year 19X3/X4)

Heading	Basis	Budget £000	General surgery Units	General surgery £000	General medicine Units	General medicine £000	Child health Units	Child health £000	Gynaecology Units	Gynaecology £000	Respiratory medicine Units	Respiratory medicine £000	Totals Units	Totals £000
Medical	Direct assignment	1 580		300		370		310		310		290		1 580
Ward nursing	Direct assignment	5 200		1250		1300		980		820		850		5 200
Theatres	Theatre hours	700	800	560					200	140			1 000	700
Drugs	Issues (£10 000 units)	400	10	100	12	120	6	60	5	50	7	70	40	400
Pharmacy	Prorata to issues	120	10	30	12	36	6	18	5	15	7	21	40	120
Radiology	Weighted radiology units	260	25 000	65	30 000	78	15 000	39	10 000	26	20 000	52	100 000	260
Pathology	Weighted pathology units	660	12 000	200	6 600	110	4 800	80	7 200	120	9 000	150	39 600	660
Catering	Patient days	480	18 000	120	15 000	100	12 000	80	15 000	100	12 000	80	72 000	480
Management	Deaths and discharges	250	2 650	60	2 114	48	1 550	35	3 205	73	1 513	34	11 033	250
Energy	Volume	250	100	50	120	60	90	45	70	35	120	60	500	250
Capital charges	Direct assignment	100		20		25		10		15		30		100
Total		10 000		2755		2247		1657		1704		1637		10 000

Notes:
1. **Calculation method**. For each functional budget not directly assigned, the activity measure for each directorate is divided by the total activity for the function and multiplied by the total budget. For example:

Cost of catering for general surgery is (18 000/72 000) × £480 000 = £120 000.

2. **Budget make-up**. All budgets shown include staff and non-staff costs and capital charges, except for capital charges to clinical directorates which are shown separately.

It is then a matter of working through those budgets not already analysed to directorates, apportioning these costs on some sensible basis. Often there will be more than one choice, perhaps with one clearly being superior to the others. The decision as to which to use is important because it can have a major bearing on each directorate's total costs and hence on its contract prices.

Table 11.1 provides an example schedule illustrating how directorate costs might be produced from a provider's functional budgets using various cost apportionment bases. Note also how the final column provides a control total to ensure that all £10 000 000 worth of budgets are reflected in directorate costs.

Accounting for inflation

One major difference between the costs included in budgets and the costs included in contract prices is that the former normally excludes anticipated inflation for the coming year whilst the latter must include it. This is referred to as the **out-turn** position. As a result, the next stage in the pricing process is to uplift costs/budgets to incorporate anticipated staff and non-staff inflation and for any net increases expected in capital charges. The actual percentages used for the uplift are yet another crucial decision and normally there is a separate estimate for at least each of the following headings reflecting both the **part-year effect** and the **full-year effect** of inflation:

- Pay Review Body staff groups (e.g. medical, nursing)
- other staff groups
- non-staff
- capital charges.

Inflation for major non-staff headings, such as energy, drugs and rates, may be separately estimated because of their relative size.

Inflation is the one major influencing factor on costs that is totally beyond the control of local management, heightening the importance of the considerations. There are no rules as such as to how a correct set of percentages can be determined. Centrally published resource assumptions can act as a guide and the Pay Review Body awards may even have been announced, but a whole range of other factors ranging from the general economic climate, the strength of the pound, interest rates and economic trends must be taken into consideration. In the end it amounts to a combination of experience and luck.

Table 11.2 illustrates the position when the example budgets have been uplifted for anticipated inflation (the 'basis' column has been omitted). Note in particular:

- How the overall percentage increase for each function was determined – this is called the 'effective increase'. An alternative, and much better, method would be to show the staff and non-staff budgets for each department separately on the schedule.
- The overall effective increase for the provider is 4.42%, but for each directorate the figure is different. This is because of the different relative weighting of costs.

Table 11.2 Analysis of provider's total budgets by directorate, uplifted for estimated inflation (financial year 19X3/X4)

Heading	Budget £000	Inflation	Uplifted £000	General surgery Units	£000	General medicine Units	£000	Child health Units	£000	Gynaecology Units	£000	Respiratory medicine Units	£000	Totals Units	£000
Medical	1 580	5.00%	1 659		315		389		326		326		305		1 659
Ward nursing	5 200	5.00%	5 460		1313		1365		1029		861		893		5 460
Theatres	700	3.21%	722	800	578					200	144			1 000	722
Drugs	400	3.25%	413	10	103	12	124	6	62	5	52	7	72	40	413
Pharmacy	120	4.00%	125	10	31	12	37	6	19	5	16	7	22	40	125
Radiology	260	3.69%	270	25 000	67	30 000	81	15 000	40	10 000	27	20 000	54	100 000	270
Pathology	660	3.47%	683	12 000	207	6 600	114	4 800	83	7 200	124	9 000	155	39 600	683
Catering	480	3.31%	496	18 000	124	15 000	103	12 000	83	15 000	103	12 000	83	72 000	496
Management	250	3.63%	259	2 650	62	2 114	49	1 550	36	3 206	75	1 583	37	11 103	259
Energy	250	1.63%	254	100	51	120	61	90	46	70	36	120	61	500	254
Capital charges	100	2.00%	102		20		26		10		15		31		102
Total	10 000		10 442		2871		2349		1733		1778		1711		10 442
Pre-inflation totals (Table 11.1)					2755		2247		1657		1704		1637		10 000
Overall percentage increase					4.22%		4.53%		4.59%		4.38%		4.53%		4.42%

Percentage increases assumed:

	Full-year effect	Part-year effect
Pay Review Body staff groups	5.00%	5.00%
Other staff groups	4.00%	4.00%
Drugs	6.00%	3.25%
Energy	3.00%	1.63%
Other non-staff	4.00%	2.17%
Capital charges	3.70%	2.00%

Percentages shown against each line reflect the overall effect in functional department, which will depend upon the mix of staff and non-staff. To illustrate:

Pathology department:

	Budget £000	Inflation	Uplifted £000
Pay Review Body staff	60	5.00%	63
Other staff	380	4.00%	395
Non-staff	200	2.17%	204
Capital charges	20	2.00%	21
	660		683
Overall effective percentage			3.47%

Note: Some totals are rounded.

Accounting for SIFTR

A final major adjustment to the figures may be required in the case of providers with teaching or research responsibilities. It is recognized that, because of the costs incurred by training undergraduate medical students and undertaking approved research, their prices are higher than would otherwise be the case, potentially placing them at a disadvantage when compared to non-teaching neighbours. An additional allocation known as SIFTR (Service Increment for Teaching and Research) was, for many years, provided to teaching health authorities to meet these costs. This entitlement has been retained in their transfer to the purchasing role, with the intention that it fund the additional costs included by teaching providers in their prices. The best policy from a provider's view is to obtain SIFTR as a 'block contract'. The block amount received can then be deducted from the bottom line of the pricing schedule in line with the associated cost incurrence at the end of the exercise – in effect treating it as a subsidy. The alternative of relying on purchasers to pass on SIFTR through general contract prices is inevitably more risky in the longer term.

Analysis by patient type

Having determined total directorate or specialty costs, including inflation and ad-justed for SIFTR if appropriate, the same principles may be applied for analysis be-tween in-patient, out-patient, day-case and day-care treatments and stays and then for any further analysis to a lower level, such as sub-specialty, DRG or procedure.

The intention is to strike a proper balance between too broad and too narrow an approach to contract pricing given the information, information technology and operational systems available. As a starting point, selective refinement of contract prices within a directorate or specialty is a sensible development, particularly where specialized and/or relatively low-volume, high-cost treatments are provided. In such instances a zero-based 'bottom-up' approach can usefully be adopted, assuming that the relevant functional and departmental activity/workload associated with the pro-vision of these services can clearly be determined. Also, as stressed above, patients receiving these specialized treatments need to be properly identified and recorded, and if large sums of income are at stake it is advisable for the clinical staff to be directly involved in this process. This is even more crucial if treatments are chargeable as elective extra contractual referrals. Costs incorporated in selective procedural prices by this means must not be included a second time when deriving prices for any other contract activity in the directorate or specialty.

Returning to the pricing schedule, it is now possible to calculate individual contract prices and analyse anticipated income by purchaser. Table 11.3 sets out the anti-cipated contracts analysed by purchaser.

It is on the activity shown in Table 11.3 that all costs have been based. The first point to notice is that separate contracts are expected for in-patient and out-patient activity. This requires a further analysis of costs in those directorates, using the same basic principles, between those incurred treating in-patients and those incurred treating out-patients. The results are as shown in Table 11.4.

With all the required information now available, individual contract prices can be determined by dividing the costs by the associated level of patient activity, including any planned or anticipated ECR activity, to derive an average (standard) cost per

Table 11.3 Analysis of anticipated activity by purchaser (financial year 19X3/X4)

	General surgery		General medicine		Child health		Gynaecology		Respiratory medicine		Totals	
	D & D	Out-pat.	D & D	Out-pat.	D & D	Out-pat.	D & D	Out-pat.	D & D	Out-pat.	D & D	Out-pat.
Purchaser A	750	450	700	0	700	0	500	0	550	300	3200	750
Purchaser B	100	60	80	0	50	0	100	0	150	120	480	180
Purchaser C	50	30	70	0	0	0	70	0	30	20	220	50
Purchaser D	30	10	0	0	0	0	0	0	10	5	40	15
Purchaser E	20	0	0	0	0	0	30	0	10	5	60	5
	950	550	850	0	750	0	700	0	750	450	4000	1000

Notes:
1. In-patient activity expressed in deaths and discharges (D & D).
2. Out-patient activity expressed in new referrals.

Table 11.4 Analysis of directorate costs between in-patient and out-patient interventions

	General surgery £000	Respiratory medicine £000
In-patients	2300	1300
Out-patients	571	411
	2871	1711

unit of activity. The total expected income from each purchaser, whether from contracts or from ECR billing, can then be determined by multiplying the standard cost per unit by the number of units. Both of these steps are shown in Table 11.5.

Once the total cost per directorate/specialty has been obtained and analysed by patient type, contract prices can be calculated for different currencies. For example, if there are large variations in length of stay in a particular contract it may be decided to contract on a cost-per-patient-day basis. Whilst this will not change the total income received it may result in a change of analysis by purchaser, as illustrated in Table 11.6 for general surgery.

Table 11.6 Analysis of comparative income expectations using different currencies (financial year 19X3/X4)

General surgery in-patients:

	D & D (a)	ALOS (b)	Total I/P days (a × b)	Cost per I/P day £	Revised income £
Purchaser A	750	4.8	3600	484	1 743 158
Purchaser B	100	5.4	540	484	261 474
Purchaser C	50	6.2	310	484	150 105
Purchaser D	30	6.0	180	484	87 158
Purchaser E	20	6.0	120	484	58 105
	950	5.0	4750		2 300 000

Notes:
1. D & D = deaths and discharges.
2. ALOS = average length of stay.
3. Cost per in-patient day = (2 300 000/4750) = £484.
4. Total income per purchaser = Cost per day × Total I/P days.

Note how the change in currency has impacted upon individual purchasers. If patient days is used as the currency less income is expected from Purchaser A, but more is expected from each of the others. Therefore it is important to ensure that there is a clear understanding of expected contract currencies when undertaking this stage of the pricing exercise.

Finalizing price and income levels

Having calculated the contract prices, the agreeing of formal contracts with each purchaser can begin. The key areas of discussion include:

Table 11.5 Calculation of contract prices and analysis of income by purchaser (financial year 19X3/X4)

Costs and activity summary

	General surgery		General medicine		Child health		Gynaecology		Respiratory medicine		Total		Grand total
	In-pat.	Out-pat.	In-pat.	Out-pat.	In-pat.	Out-pat.	In-pat.	Out-pat.	In-pat.	Out-pat.	In-pat.	Out-pat.	
Costs (Tables 11.2 and 11.4)	2 300 000	571 000	2 349 000		1 733 000		1 778 000		1 300 000	411 000	9 460 000	982 000	10 442 000
Activity (Table 11.3)	950	550	850		750		700		750	450	4 000	1 000	
Contract price – £	2421	1038	2764		2311		2540		1733	913	2365	982	

Income by purchaser (analysis as per Table 11.3)

	General surgery		General medicine		Child health		Gynaecology		Respiratory medicine		Totals		
	D & D £	Out-pat. £	D & D £	Out-pat. £	D & D £	Out-pat. £	D & D £	Out-pat. £	D & D £	Out-pat. £	D & D £	Out-pat. £	Grand total £
Purchaser A	1 815 789	467 182	1 934 471	0	1 617 467	0	1 270 000	0	953 333	274 000	7 591 060	741 182	8 332 242
Purchaser B	242 105	62 291	221 082	0	115 533	0	254 000	0	260 000	109 600	1 092 721	171 891	1 264 612
Purchaser C	121 053	31 145	193 447	0	0	0	177 800	0	52 000	18 267	544 300	49 412	593 712
Purchaser D	72 632	10 382	0	0	0	0	0	0	17 333	4 567	89 965	14 948	104 913
Purchaser E	48 421	0	0	0	0	0	76 200	0	17 333	4 567	141 954	4 567	146 521
	2 300 000	571 000	2 349 000	0	1 733 000	0	1 778 000	0	1 300 000	411 000	9 460 000	982 000	10 442 000

Notes:
1. Contract price for general surgery in-patients = (2 300 000/950) = £2421.
2. Income expected from Purchaser A for general surgery in-patients = (2421 × 750) = £1 815 789.
3. Some totals are rounded.

- contract types (block, cost and volume, cost per case);
- contract currencies;
- contract activity volumes;
- activity to be charged on an ECR basis (i.e. requiring prior authorization);
- price, with particular reference to:
  - assumed inflation increases
  - any new developments included
  - cost improvement programme proposals;

- quality standards – the definition of a price includes reference to a 'specified' level of activity. This does not mean just the normal explicit measure of patient volumes agreed for each contract (quantity), but would also include any measures concerned with the quality of provision. Quality has a cost and this too must be reflected in the price.

Some of these items are key variables in the pricing process, particularly:

- planned activity level
- planned associated costs
- estimated inflation
- cost apportionment basis.

Contract negotiation and finalization involves a series of meetings with each of the different purchasers in turn. Any adjustment to the key variables used in the contract pricing process affects one or more contract prices and, depending upon the mix of activity purchased, may affect some or all purchasers. If a change in the variables is required or requested by a purchaser part way through this series of meetings, there is a distinct possibility that this will impact on the contracts already tentatively agreed. The impact of a change in each variable can now be considered in turn.

Planned activity level

This is the variable that is most likely to cause problems in practice. The budget setting exercise requires an identification of anticipated outcome/output in order that an assessment of required resource consumption can be undertaken. Because of the possibility of actual contract activity differing from budgeted contract activity, an assessment has to be made of the additional resources that will be consumed if additional work is undertaken, or the resources that will not be consumed if less work is undertaken. This is referred to as cost behaviour analysis and involves an application of the standard costing techniques.

The greater part of a provider's costs are fixed and are absorbed across anticipated patient activity levels. If the actual patient activity is less than anticipated then not all of the fixed costs will be recovered and a deficit will occur. The provider theoretically then has two choices: either reduce costs, or absorb all costs in the lower activity. By the very definition of fixed costs the first of these choices is not possible in the shorter term, so the fixed costs have to be absorbed across the reduced activity level, thereby increasing the contract price. This affects not just the purchaser requiring a

Contracts for 750 respiratory medicine in-patients are expected for 19X3/X4, as analysed in Table 11.3. The build-up of total anticipated costs is analysed and the following split is determined:

	£000
Variable costs	375
Fixed costs	925
	1300

Cost per case:

	£
Variable cost per patient = £375 000/750	500
Fixed cost per patient = £925 000/750	1233
Total cost (as per Table 11.5)	1733

During contract negotiations Purchaser B indicates that they have a requirement for 50 patients, instead of the 150 they required last year and originally thought that they would require again this year, thereby reducing total activity from 750 to 650.
The revised costs for this service are then as follows:

	£000
Variable costs (£500 × 650)	325
Fixed costs	925
	1250

Cost per case:

	£
Variable cost per patient	500
Fixed cost per patient = £925 000/650	1423
Total cost (as per Table 11.5)	1923

Figure 11.1 Impact of revised activity levels on contract prices.

reduced level of activity, but all purchasers purchasing that type of care. This is illustrated in Figure 11.1, using respiratory medicine in-patients as the example.

In Figure 11.1, the price per in-patient day has increased from £1733 to £1923 simply because less activity is required. This increase can be explained by the fact that fixed costs equal to £1233 × 100 = £123 300 which would have been recovered by those 100 patients now have to be recovered by the remaining activity of 650

Respiratory medicine in-patients	Revised activity	Revised price £	Revised income £	Originally expected income £	Difference £
Purchaser A	550	1923	1 057 692	953 333	104 359
Purchaser B	50	1923	96 154	260 000	(163 846)
Purchaser C	30	1923	57 692	52 000	5692
Purchaser D	10	1923	19 231	17 333	1897
Purchaser E	10	1923	19 231	17 333	1897
	650		1 250 000	1 300 000	(50 000)

Note: Totals are rounded.

Figure 11.2 Impact of revised pricing on income by purchaser (financial year 19X3/X4).

patients, i.e. an increase of £123 300/650 = £190. Figure 11.2 sets out the impact of this upon each purchaser.

It can be seen from Figure 11.2 that if this volume adjustment were actioned in this way Purchaser B's costs are reduced far more than by the variable cost saving of 100 patients × £500 = £50 000. The redistribution of fixed costs has increased the benefit to Purchaser B at the expense of the other purchasers. This would inevitably cause problems if contracts had already been agreed with any of these.

If this reduced activity requirement has been known well in advance of the exercise being undertaken, the contract prices offered would automatically be based upon the lower level of 650 cases. This can still potentially cause problems because, for example, Purchaser A may then decide that the price of £1923 is higher than expected and even uncompetitive. Even if the price is still competitive, it may be more than can be afforded. Coupled with that, most purchasers requiring the same number of cases this year as they did last year undoubtedly expect to pay no more than that paid last year plus inflation.

To live within whatever total amount has been allocated to secure respiratory medicine contracts, the purchaser may decide to reduce the number of cases required such that the lower activity level multiplied by the contract price equals total funding available. This then exacerbates the situation as the fixed costs then have to be spread over even fewer cases, thereby forcing the cost per case upwards, making the price even less attractive. At the extreme there is the danger that price spiralling may occur until purchasers decide not to purchase any such activity from the provider, leaving the fixed costs totally unrecovered. These costs then have to be recovered by including them in contracts for other types of patient activity, with exactly the same danger of the spiral effect occurring there.

Such a situation is of concern to providers and purchasers alike, and there are a number of devices that those more short-sighted or inexperienced in the role of procurement may try. In particular, it is in the interest of all parties to ensure that a single purchaser does not try to agree a contract at an activity level substantially lower than historical referral patterns simply to benefit in the way illustrated above, with the intention of then retaining the historical referral levels and paying for the difference between contracted activity and actual activity at the end of the year at marginal cost.

Planned associated costs

If a single major purchaser indicates that a particular contract price is too high it may be agreed to revisit the costing exercise to determine whether costs can be reduced. Possibly certain developments have been included within the price that the purchaser is unwilling to approve. Cost reduction is most unlikely to be of a form that affects the patients of only one purchaser. For example, if the contract price included a proposed increase to the staff establishment on a ward by 1.00 WTE as a service development, the withdrawal of this proposal reduces the cost of treating all patients and so reduces the contract price for all purchasers. Therefore, assuming that the 'avoidance of cross-subsidization' rule is being applied correctly, what may at first appear to be a small cost reduction to satisfy one purchaser may turn out to require a substantial amount of cost saving to be achieved.

Estimated inflation

Similar difficulties arise with disagreements regarding the level of inflation included within contract pricing calculations. For example, one purchaser may try to insist that the correct level of non-staff inflation to be included is 2%, when all others are happy to accept 3%. There is no straightforward means by which differential inflation rates can be applied on a purchaser basis and so, unless some rather complex weighting calculations are used, such a reduction if agreed would benefit all purchasers in proportion.

Cost apportionment basis

If it is attempted to reduce a contract price by means of apportioning indirect costs and/or fixed overheads on a different basis, it is likely that a number of other prices, if not all, will be affected. The impact on each purchaser of this revision is totally dependent upon the relative volumes concerned.

Summary

It is apparent from this brief consideration that a change in any of the key variables, or a change in one of the other variables such as contract currency, impacts on many or all purchasers, the full extent depending upon the relative mix of activity being purchased. This emphasizes just how crucial an accurate assessment and agreement of each of these factors early on in the pricing process really is. It is often best practice first to discuss such variables with the main purchaser(s) to obtain some broad degree of acceptance of the principles that will be employed.

These variables present provider and purchaser alike with a number of risks, but they furnish the provider with flexibility to come up with a range of prices for a particular service. Underestimating activity levels or overestimating costs and inflation pushes prices up, and vice versa. Too high a price may turn away business, but too low a price may end up under-recovering costs. Purchasers have a finite sum available and winning business in one area may mean losing it in another with no net gain. The final decision on pricing is inevitably down to local experience. At this level, and given the huge sums of money potentially at stake, financial management becomes more like risk management.

Major factors influencing contract price

The main variables influencing the contract price are discussed above. However, in terms of price calculation it is highly likely that, overall, the cost apportionment method is the major determinant of costs and hence prices, much more so than any direct cost allocation. If a particular contract price looks high, it does not automatically mean that the provider is less efficient. It may, for example, simply be that indirect costs and overheads are apportioned in a different way, a way that could be less correct, or more correct. Where such costs form a large part of total cost, even small changes in the apportionment basis can cause major swings in price.

Similarly, a high proportion of capital charges in the total cost can easily conceal or distort operational efficiencies. This is a particular area of difficulty where very old buildings occupy sites of high land value, or supply what might be termed 'low-tech' services. There are wide variations across the country when expressed as a percentage of total costs.

This is not to say that providers can defend any high price with such excuses. Refinement of the costing and pricing process will, over time, reduce such distortions, but probably never remove them, especially given that costing can be considered as much an art as a science.

Costing and pricing by diagnosis related groups – the future?

Despite the fact that much effort has been expended in refining costing and pricing processes within the NHS there is still much work yet to be done, including establishing the level at which contracts commonly should be priced. In the 1980s much interest was shown in the diagnosis related group (DRG) approach to patient grouping. The attraction stemmed in part from a recognition of the benefits of adopting a recognized and thoroughly researched system such as DRGs. In particular it was seen as allowing cost comparisons between service providers for the same patient grouping, although it must be accepted that such comparisons cannot be meaningful without knowledge of the cost apportionment techniques employed. Whilst DRGs gained much favour early on in the formal Resource Management

Initiative, and are still perhaps the most well-known technique, their level of acceptance is, at the time of writing, perhaps considerably less than originally forecast.

The introduction of contracting has furthered the debate over the value of DRGs in the NHS. Some associate the RMI with DRGs, and DRGs with contracts. However, there has not been any decision to make DRGs an essential part of any RMI system nor any suggestion that DRGs must form the basis of contracts. This latter point ties in with the fact that DRGs play no part in the funding of purchasers, for whom weighted capitation will continue to be used.

DRG is a costing technique which can usefully be applied to deriving clinical budgets, although it was never specifically designed for this purpose. If it is eventually to be accepted as the common basis for contract pricing, it must be seen as representing the approach to patient grouping that best combines an avoidance of broad and unrepresentative averaging techniques with an acceptance that some form of patient grouping is unavoidable. Currently, the focus appears to be more towards costing by procedures, especially as GP fundholder contract prices are required at this level. The continual increase in technological capabilities may yet see the 'procedure' oust the DRG as the common contract currency of the future.

Conclusion

Contract pricing in the NHS generally adopts the top-down costing approach, primarily due to a lack of the sophistications necessary to apply properly the bottom-up method. Whilst this is simpler, quicker and cheaper, the results are likely to be less accurate and hence lack credence. What has to be decided in every case is whether the extra costs incurred in refining contract prices are outweighed by the resultant benefits.

The freedom of providers to define their 'product' can lead to a lack of comparability between published contract prices. This is especially so as this freedom extends to the methods applied in apportioning the relatively large proportion of indirect and overhead costs that make up total contract costs. Capital charges are another major influence on final price. Wide variations between providers of these as a percentage of total costs means that comparisons of price will not reflect only relative operational efficiencies.

The complex impact of changes in key variables, especially when dealing with a number of major purchasers, can lead to apparent anomalies in the pricing process. Providers and purchasers have to work together to ensure that such changes do not result in a destabilization of the local market.

Questions

1. The 'bottom-up' approach to contract costing is not widely applied. Explain the reasons for this, comparing its advantages and disadvantages with the 'top-down' method.
2. What stages are there in the contract pricing process? Which are the most important, and why?
3. What are the major factors that influence cost, and hence price? Why is their influence so great?

4. To what extent are DRGs truly representative of relative resource consumption patterns, and hence cost? What alternatives are available as a basis for contracting, and what are their advantages and disadvantages?

*5. The Midgate Trust intends to produce an initial set of 19X5/X6 contract prices for discussion with purchasers. The costs and assumptions on which they are to be based are given in Tables 11.7 and 11.8.

Table 11.7 Actual costs 19X4/X5

| Dept/Directorate | Fixed costs | | Variable costs | | Total costs £000 |
	Staff £000	Non-staff £000	Staff £000	Non-staff £000	
General surgery:					
Direct costs	600	100	100	100	900
Overheads/recharges:					
Pathology	200	100	0	100	400
Radiology	150	150	0	200	500
Pharmacy	150	50	0	300	500
Works/utilities	50	100	0	50	200
Housekeeping	50	20	0	0	70
Catering	70	150	0	50	270
Management	130	30	0	0	160
	1400	700	100	800	3000
General medicine:					
Direct costs	1000	150	50	300	1500
Overheads/recharges:					
Pathology	350	200	0	150	700
Radiology	200	200	0	300	700
Pharmacy	200	100	0	400	700
Works/utilities	70	130	0	100	300
Housekeeping	50	20	0	0	70
Catering	100	180	0	70	350
Management	150	30	0	0	180
	2120	1010	50	1320	4500
Total all costs	3520	1710	150	2120	7500

Table 11.8 Interim contract pricing assumptions 19X5/X6

A. Inflation
Staff	2.50%
Non-staff	3.50%
Capital charges	4.50%

B. CIP   0.00%

C. Contract activity measured in deaths and discharges (D & D):

	General surgery	General medicine	Total
Purchaser A	3000	5300	8 300
Purchaser B	1000	2500	3 500
Purchaser C	1800	200	2 000
Purchaser D	200	0	200
	6000	8000	14 000

Notes:
- There were no non-recurring costs incurred in 19X4/X5.
- Patient activity volumes for 19X5/X6 are assumed to be identical to volumes for 19X4/X5.
- Fixed non-staff costs shown in Table 11.7 are all capital charges.
- Variable costs incurred/charged to each directorate vary directly with patient activity.

Required:
(a) Calculate the initial contract price, based on the information provided in Tables 11.7 and 11.8. Analyse the expected income by purchaser.
(b) During contract negotiations, the interim assumptions given in Table 11.8 have to be changed to those shown in Table 11.9. Calculate the combined impact of these changes on the interim 19X5/X6 contract prices and income analysis by purchaser. What do you note about the movement in total income analysis by purchaser?

Table 11.9 Actual contract pricing variables 19X5/X6

A. Inflation

Staff	2.00%
Non-staff	4.00%
Capital charges	8.00%

B. CIP*   1.00%

C. Contract activity (D & D):

	General surgery	General medicine	Total
Purchaser A	4000	5300	9 300
Purchaser B	1000	2000	3 000
Purchaser C	1800	200	2 000
Purchaser D	100	100	200
	6900	7600	14 500

*The requirement to reduce costs by 1.00% × £7 500 000 = £75 000 will be achieved through reducing the on-call pathology service provided to general surgery. Pathology staff costs, and hence recharges, will reduce by this amount (at 19X4/X5 prices). These recharges are included under the heading of Overheads/recharges: Fixed costs, Staff.

12

Financial management in the contracting environment

AIMS

The introduction of the new financial environment, based on a split between the purchasers and providers of health care, has had a major impact on both funding and management arrangements within the NHS, particularly as a result of the creation of NHS Trusts (NHSTs). The aims of this chapter are to:

- examine how the introduction of the purchaser–provider split has impacted upon approaches to resource management;
- identify how financial management can be undertaken in the contracting environment;
- provide an insight into the applicability of the formal Resource Management Initiative;
- describe the process of negotiating and subsequently controlling contracts;
- show how strategies and plans are developed;
- explain the use of service level agreements.

Background to contracting

Prior to the introduction of the system based on contracts, the funding allocation passed down through the management hierarchy to the level at which patient care was provided was based upon an incremental approach. This meant that, at its simplest, each level in the hierarchy received last year's funding, uplifted for inflation and any agreed developments. The major disadvantage of the incremental approach was that funding was provided to units without any specific indication of the patient activity levels they were expected to provide, although the intention that waiting lists should be reduced during the year might be specified as a goal. However, only where specific 'waiting list funding' was provided was there likely to be a strong link between funding and activity. Thus, specific waiting list initiatives aside, units received a fixed level of funding regardless of the number of patients treated.

Unit funding, once established, was passed to budget managers. Below the level of very senior management, unit budget managers generally had little knowledge of funding allocation issues, nor any need to gain such knowledge. What they did understand, in most units, was that the unit would be given funds based on the amount received in the previous year. This sum would then be divided up between budgets on a similar historical basis, and so, no matter how much their department's or function's workload varied due to changes in patient numbers, it was most unlikely that their budget would be varied to match. The lack of any direct link between funding and workload meant that only if developmental funding became available was it likely that additional resources could be obtained to assist in meeting the costs of related additional departmental activity. In practice, some units had introduced the concept of budget flexing as part of their overall resource management initiatives, but even these still remained constrained by the overall unit allocation and had to finance budget flexing from within this fixed amount.

A number of initiatives intended to assist the proper management of resources were introduced after the 1974 reorganization. For the most part, these were designed to improve financial management within district health authorities by focusing awareness on the relationships between activity and revenue costs at the sharp end of the Service, that is the units delivering health care. However, none of these initiatives truly addressed the anomaly that, no matter how efficient a unit became when compared to another, the traditional NHS allocation distribution method did not automatically promote redirection of funding from the less efficient to the more efficient unit to take advantage of this situation.

The policy-makers recognized that this had the potential to act as a disincentive to increased efficiency and effectiveness and that a means of rectifying this peculiarity had to be found. This problem had to be overcome in such a way that it did not destroy a most fundamental principle of the NHS, that is, NHS finance must be **equitably divided** (allocated) across the country based upon **relative demographic need**. It would not be acceptable simply to fund services geographically based upon the efficiency and effectiveness of hospitals because this would take no account of the relative needs of patients in different parts of the country. What was needed was a methodology of allocation distribution that counterbalanced the maxim of allocating funds within the Service strategically on the basis of need with that of delivering services locally with the highest possible degree of efficiency and effectiveness.

The introduction of contracting arrangements for patient care was seen as the appropriate means of achieving this aim. A clear division of responsibility was introduced between health care purchasers and health care providers, with the relationship being controlled by formal contracts. The aim of the contracting arrangements was and remains to influence financial management in a totally different way, by introducing an element of 'competition' to the health-care market so as to influence activity directly in a way that optimizes resource consumption. The specific intention is that, given a finite amount of funding, purchasers will maximize the level of care obtained for their residents by purchasing each component of their overall package of requirements from those providers offering the best value for money as represented by the best mix of quality, accessibility and price. An implicit assumption is that a greater number of patients treated equals a greater level of health benefit.

Competition between providers is intended to encourage the achievement of maximum value for money by forcing them to examine both the quality and price of their services against competitors in order to win contracts and thereby secure funding. Contracts generally relate to patient activity levels and so the advantage of this approach is seen to be that the level of funding provided is related to the number of patients treated since 'money follows the patient'.

Impact of the revised funding process

The fundamental difference to the funding process is that providers can no longer rely on receiving a volume of funds based on an historical allocation level. Instead they must look to income earned from fulfilling contracts as their main source of funding. This both provides opportunities and poses risks, and potentially, given the fact that an overall cash limit exists, for every winner under these arrangements there must be a loser. However, it can be argued that if all providers improve their efficiency and effectiveness they will not necessarily be 'losers'.

This certainly increases the importance of an awareness and understanding of both sides of the contract-focused market. Its operation must be understood not just by managers, but also all those in provider organizations influencing income earning and/or resource consumption decisions.

Income is derived from the delivery of the three types of patient contract described in an earlier chapter. A certain element of income may also be anticipated from extra contractual referrals (ECRs), particularly for acute services. Indeed, in some providers these form a significant part of total income and therefore take on a particular importance.

Prior to the introduction of contracting, cross-boundary flows of patients occurred when the residents of one DHA were treated by health care facilities of another. These patient flows were funded in the historical allocation of the DHA providing the treatment and not in the DHA where the patient lived. There was no factual link between, or monitoring of, the relationship between the volume of patient flows and the level of funding provided.

A threat that became apparent with the introduction of contracts followed the repatriation of historical cross-boundary flow allocations between DHAs. Now, each DHA receives funds to purchase care for their resident population wherever they are treated, i.e. money follows the patient.

In the early years of contracting the temptation for some DHAs was to spend newly acquired funding in their own DMUs, rather than to maintain traditional referral patterns. For some providers, especially centres of excellence which drew their patients from a wide geographical area, cross-boundary flows were a significant percentage of their activity and hence income. Given the predominantly fixed cost structure in the short term, any reduction in long-established funding levels would result in overspends until costs could be matched to income levels. The converse of placing sudden demands for increased activity upon other providers could have resulted in the inappropriate use of limited resources. For example, if a provider had for many years treated a small number of haematology cases and suddenly had dramatically to increase throughput, it may not have the physical or technical capability and would need to invest in additional beds, equipment and suitably trained staff. This transition would be difficult to accomplish in an efficient manner in a short timescale.

Thus in the early years of contracting it was essential that the introduction of flows of cash as well as patients did not destabilize the health market. Due to these difficulties central guidance and encouragement ensured financial neutrality during the early years. However, the market has seen the formation of 'purchasing consortia', which are made up of the two types of purchasing authorities, namely DHAs and FHSAs. Such consortia may compose two or more DHAs or a DHA and an FHSA or a group of DHAs and FHSAs. Some DHAs have simply amalgamated, to form 'commissioning agencies'. At the same time there has been a substantial increase in the number of NHS trusts. These developments have weakened previous DMU loyalties and the development of purchasing consortia−trust relationships now normally pays little regard to past purchasing patterns, thereby increasing threats and opportunities to providers.

The changes which have already taken place, and those in prospect, make proper financial management of both income and expenditure absolutely essential to the continuing operation of the provider. Indeed, ongoing financial viability is a key prerequisite prior to the formation of a trust. Trusts must also be able to demonstrate ongoing financial viability through the preparation of annual financial plans.

Sound financial management requires sound planning and control. Planning has always been important in the NHS, but its importance is now paramount. Providers now have to plan ahead to determine not only how they intend to spend their funding but, more importantly, how they are going to acquire it in the first place. Those involved with financial management at all levels in the organization must be aware of both sides of this important equation. This far more business-like approach requires an enormous amount of work but has brought to NHS operational planning a far greater clarity. Arguably, it has done more to force the involvement of clinical staff in the management process, in contrast to what was more of an encouragement of such involvement in previous initiatives. Clinical staff play a key role in assisting with the development of a provider's business strategy and now influence not only the spending (expenditure) side of the equation, but also the funding (income) side.

Strategies and plans

The direct link between funding and patient activity levels has the consequence that financial plans must inevitably take into account patient activity plans, and be dependent upon such plans. Therefore the starting point in the planning process must now be a clear definition of planned patient activity for the period. Such plans have, in turn, to be converted into contracts that will be both appealing and satisfactory to purchaser organizations and, equally importantly, that are affordable by them.

This requires a clearly defined business strategy which identifies, amongst other things:

- planned patient levels, which in turn requires an assessment of anticipated demand, at an appropriate level of detail;

- anticipated costs and hence desired income from that level of activity;
- planned application of that funding across budgets;
- the level of capital investment, re-investment, or disinvestment required, and the revenue consequences of these plans.

The first of these requirements is often referred to as forming the provider's contracting strategy, whilst the second and third requirements are often described as the financial strategy with the fourth as the investment or capital strategy.

Plans and strategies must obviously relate to a defined period and are required for:

- the short term, generally one financial year or less
- the medium term, one to three years
- the long term, three to five years or even more.

Proper financial management requires, and benefits from, an awareness of these strategies and plans and a particular understanding of their interrelationships and their relevance towards and impact on operational matters. Figure 12.1 identifies these relationships.

The short-term contracting strategy is set out in each provider's annual business plan. This has to specify the proposed activities of the provider for the coming year, and their relevance to contracting aspirations and intentions. It should also integrate directly with capital investment proposals and with the provider's financial plans. The threats and risks to the provider stemming from any variations to anticipated

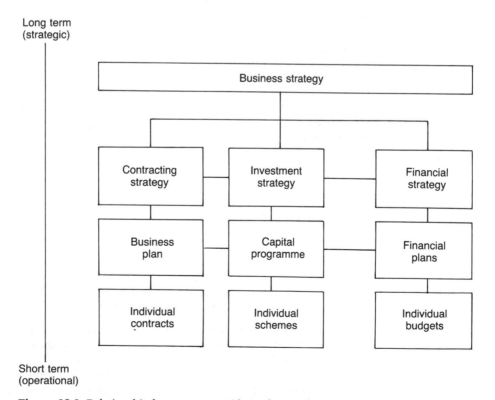

Figure 12.1 Relationship between a provider's plans and strategies.

contracted activity should be identified, together with their impact on investment and income. The opportunities open to undertake additional work either from agreeing additional contracts or from non-recurring waiting-list type initiatives must also be included.

The investment strategy, upon which the business plan relies, is reflected in the provider's annual capital programme, recognizing that some individual schemes may cover more than one financial year. In practice the annual investment programme may be published as part of that year's business plan.

The short-term financial plans encapsulated in the financial strategy are expressed in monetary terms in the detailed revenue and income budgets agreed with budget managers. It is possible to budget to hold some sums in reserve, and these can be general, specific or for anticipated inflation. During the year, the balances held in reserve can be fed into the budget control system as enhancements to existing budgets.

Negotiating contracts

The provider organization is almost totally reliant upon income from contracts negotiated. It is possible that some income is not reliant on contracts; for example, interest on investments may be earned or providers with acknowledged teaching or research responsibilities receive SIFTR funding. Even with these exemptions, until contract negotiations are complete, the provider is not guaranteed a level of income sufficient to support its full range of activities. As a result, contract negotiation is of prime importance.

In the earlier days of contracting it was common for purchasers to agree with a provider a single block 'contract' for a range of services, sometimes with an 'indicative' volume against each major specialty group, or each chargeable procedure for GP fundholders. This contract contained either a single price for the total activity or an 'indicative' price for each specialty/chargeable procedure. The contracting process is now becoming more refined, and a disaggregation of contracts down to and below specialty level has developed and true cost and volume contracts are increasingly common.

The next stage, that of achieving meaningful cost per case type contracting, is a much greater step but one for which those providers with the more sophisticated resource management systems are well placed to take to some extent or other, should they and their purchasers agree this as the way forward. However, because of differential rates of development of the contracting process at the local level, there can be different understandings as to how exactly a 'contract' is defined. The definition is important because there are a number of key factors within the contract negotiation process which have to be agreed with each different purchaser and which impact on the contract pricing methodology. These are:

- the **form** of contract to be struck: block, cost and volume, cost per case;
- the grouping **level** at which contracts are to be struck such as: specialty, sub-specialty, DRG, or procedure;
- the **type** of contracts to be struck: in-patients, out-patients, day cases, day care, or some combination of these, for example in-patient and out-patient combined;
- the **currency** to be used – alternative measures are available: deaths and dis-

charges, patient days, total out-patient attendances, new out-patient attendances, or consultant episodes;
- the **nature** of the intervention: emergency, urgent or elective.

A contract can be defined as an agreement between two parties whereby a discrete activity or amount of work is undertaken for a specified price. In ideal circumstances, this means that for each purchaser there is a different contract for each type of activity for each different grouping at the level chosen. This can be illustrated by assuming that all contracts are struck at a specialty level, in which case each of the following would be considered as a contract:

- Purchaser A:
  - General surgery in-patients
  - General surgery out-patients
  - General surgery day cases
  - Thoracic surgery in-patients
  - Dermatology out-patients
    etc.
- Purchaser B:
  - General surgery in-patients
  - General surgery out-patients
  - General surgery day cases
  - Thoracic surgery in-patients
  - Dermatology out-patients
    etc.

However, if Purchaser C is a GP fundholder, then the requirements are expressed in terms of procedures:

- Purchaser C:
  - Procedure 41
  - Procedure 62
    etc.

In practice a provider may agree some contracts at one level, for example specialty, but others at a different level. The latter case is likely to apply in the case of highly specialized and/or high-cost interventions which may be agreed at sub-specialty or DRG level.

In addition to routine contracts, a provider is also likely to earn other income through the treatment of extra contractual referrals (ECRs). The assumed level of ECRs, because of their contribution to fixed costs, can have a significant impact on overall contract prices. When constructing a business strategy for a particular year a provider may assume a certain level of ECR income, often based upon historical trends adjusted for anticipated or known changes. This can be a relatively significant source of income for some providers, whilst for others it can be very minor.

One further factor to appreciate is that the centrally provided contract pricing rules clearly state that all fixed costs must be recovered by the planned activity levels without any cross-subsidization between contracts. Where 'unplanned' activity, which was not included at the time of calculating contract prices, is undertaken, it can only be charged for at marginal costs, that is the overheads that should already have been recovered via the main contracts cannot be charged for a second time. Such unplanned work may arise through an agreement with a purchaser to treat more patients than originally contracted for, or to undertake special waiting list initiatives. The marginal prices of such extra work may be discussed with purchasers at the time of main contract negotiation and may form an integral part of the contract. The identification of marginal costs is not only important for pricing additional activity; contracts may also use it to value agreed income reductions to reflect any shortfall in achievement.

Managing contracts

The level and type of contract struck both have a major impact on the way in which contracts are subsequently managed. The lower the level at which contracts are struck the more detailed the contract pricing exercise has to be in order to determine prices, which are based on cost, at this level. This does not cause a major problem because the annual contract pricing exercise is fairly straightforward. The more complex part is ensuring that information is available to manage at the required level on a month-to-month and even day-to-day basis. This has major repercussions both on the finance function which has to present financial information, and on the activity recording side which has to ensure that systems exist to record activity at the contracted level.

The financial and activity recording can both cause major problems. However, these are less substantial on the financial side as the financial systems, particularly ledger systems and financial reporting systems, are already fairly well established. A number of sites are also fairly well advanced in terms of implementing an RMI case mix management system which provides further information. It tends to be the patient recording side which gives providers the greatest difficulties. A number of approaches have been developed since the inception of contracting, some based around manual systems whilst others are based around computer systems. The computer systems range from the adaptation of mainframe systems to allow recording of contract detail, down to purpose built microcomputer systems.

Service level agreements

The need to understand the contracting environment and to appreciate resource management and financial management in the contracting environment is applicable not only to those dealing with patient contracts, such as clinical directors, locality managers, senior managers and those directly assisting in the process. Those responsible for the day-to-day management of services directly providing patient care, such as nursing staff and medical staff, are also reliant upon support from other departments or directorates and so need to appreciate the financial structure within which they work.

All specialties require a great number of support services such as: catering, housekeeping and portering, energy and utilities, and linen, and the majority of specialties also require assistance from other support departments such as pharmacy, ECG, lung function, and pathology. Greater complexity occurs where support departments themselves use the services of other support departments; for example, the catering department requires housekeeping services, and the housekeeping department requires energy and utilities. Ultimately all services provided within a unit/trust assist in the delivery of patient care, although some can be more directly identifiable to patient level than others.

It is highly likely that those responsible for managing support areas are different from those managing the specialties requiring their services. Very often those responsible for managing departments are not the same as those responsible for taking the decisions that result in resources being consumed within a department. It has to be recognized, however, that it would be managerially impossible for clinical directors or their equivalents to attempt to manage on a day-to-day basis all services required to run a hospital. There is no specific demarcation at which a differentiation can be made between a service that could sensibly be managed by a clinical director and one that could not, as this depends entirely on local circumstances and preferences. There are some services, such as catering, grounds and gardens, and works maintenance, that no clinical director would wish to take managerial responsibility for on a day-to-day basis. Other cases are more borderline, for example pharmacy and some of the other technical support departments, and it is common for some, or all, of these to be managed by one or more directorate. Out-patient departments, admissions departments and day case units are additional examples where it is possible to identify likely control by a clinical director. Irrespective of the manner of control, a means has to be found of overcoming the recognized problems of a budget being managed by one individual whilst other individuals make the decisions as to resource consumption levels chargeable against that budget.

Whilst there may be local variations, particularly as to name, a common means of overcoming this problem is by the setting of 'service level agreements' or 'internal contracts'. As the name implies these are agreements between departments and directorates (or between departments and other departments) to provide a certain level of service for an agreed price. The calculation of this price uses the same principles applied when calculating the patient contract prices, and all the principles discussed in determining patient contract prices can be applied for the calculation of prices for internal service level agreements. Therefore such techniques and principles are of particular interest to all budget managers and to all those responsible for delivering a certain level of service.

The service level agreements reflect the two important concerns in the overall delivery of a service:

- **Management of supply** ensures the availability of the service and that the service is **provided** in an efficient and effective manner. This is concerned with the inputs to the function and their relationship with its output.
- **Management of demand** ensures the efficient and effective **consumption** of the resultant outputs.

To illustrate, it is the professional and managerial responsibility of a clinical director of radiology to ensure that the expected range of radiological examinations and tests are undertaken when requested by medical colleagues. Furthermore, these requests must be correctly performed in an efficient and effective manner. It is the professional responsibility of the clinical director of general surgery to ensure that all necessary examinations are requested for patients under the care of the directorate. It is the managerial responsibility to ensure that no unnecessary examinations are undertaken.

This approach, when properly applied, overcomes the problem of mismatch between control of, and responsibility for, clinically demand-led budgets. If financial problems arise, any mismanagement of supply or demand is clearly highlighted by a variance analysis.

Conclusion

The understanding of resource consumption emphasized in the past decade now needs to be complemented by a thorough grasp of the means by which funding is made available at all levels in the organization. Tight expenditure controls are of little benefit if funding due is not sought, or is lost, through a lack of understanding of the contracting process.

Questions

1. The introduction of the purchaser/provider split and contracting arrangements is considered a major change in the funding allocation philosophy. To what extent is this true for purchasers and for providers? What are the advantages and disadvantages both of this new approach and of the methodology it replaced?
2. 'NHS funding must be distributed so as to ensure equity of provision.' 'NHS funding must be distributed so as to ensure maximum efficiency and effectiveness.'

   What potential difficulties are there in reconciling these two statements and how and to what extent can they be overcome? Does ensuring equity of provision mean equality of provision?
3. Assume that within a region there are:

   - four purchasing authorities: North, South, West, East;
   - five single-hospital acute trusts: North, South, West 1, West 2, East;
   - two GP fundholding practices: West, South.

   The relative geographical positions of each hospital and GPFH within the region is as shown on the map in Figure 12.2 with the dotted lines setting out the catchment areas for each of the four purchasers.

   Table 12.1 identifies the distribution of contract income for 19X3/X4 between providers, and the source of that income by purchaser on the basis of signed contracts.

   All trusts provide similar services including general surgery and general medicine. ECR income is earned by each trust from other purchasers immediately outside the regional boundary.

   The ECR reserve is held by each purchaser to meet the cost of emergency and approved elective treatment. Any year-end underspending against this reserve is projected at the end of December each year and used to fund waiting-list initiatives in general surgery and general medicine.

   Two new fundholding practices have been approved for 19X4/X5 situated at positions 'A' and 'B' on the map. Their budgets, which will be deducted from the allocation of the host purchaser, are expected to be as follows:

	£000
GPFH A	800
GPFH B	600

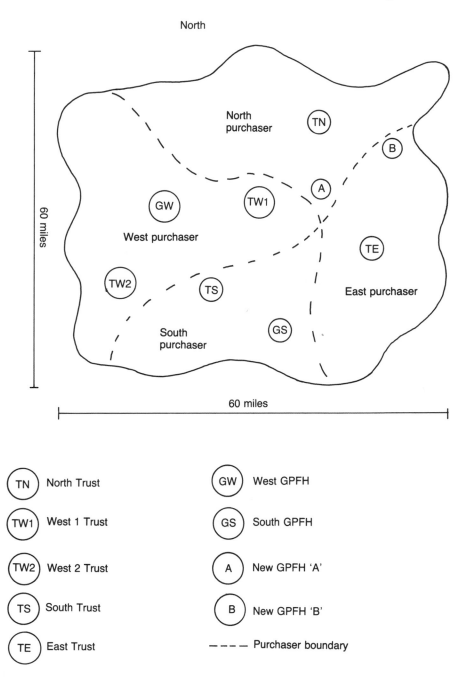

Figure 12.2 Relative geographical locations of hospitals and GPFHs in a region.

What are the current threats and opportunities to each trust? What factors will be taken into account when planning for 19X4/X5 and beyond? How and where can the information required to support the contracting, financial and investment strategies be obtained?

Table 12.1 Distribution of contract income between providers 19X13/X14

	North Trust £000	South Trust £000	West 1 Trust £000	West 2 Trust £000	East Trust £000	ECR reserve £000	Total £000
North purchaser	34 000	4 000	400	20	80	500	39 000
South purchaser	600	64 350	50	300	0	700	66 000
West purchaser	2 000	11 800	26 000	26 000	3 000	200	69 000
East purchaser	1 000	650	1 000	500	21 700	150	25 000
GPFH West	10	20	350	350	0	70	800
GPFH East	0	320	0	0	260	20	600
ECRs	160	1 060	120	120	140		1 600
	37 770	82 200	27 920	27 290	25 180	1 640	202 000

4. 'In a competitive environment there must be winners and losers.' Is this true, and if so, under what circumstances? Is it possible that all can be winners, or even all can be losers?

5. Service level agreements, otherwise known as internal contracts, are one means of dividing the management of the supply of a function from the management of the demand for it. Explain and illustrate. What alternative approaches are available and what are their relative pros and cons?

13

Performance recording and reporting

AIMS

Management in the NHS, as with any organization, is a continuous process that can be considered as taking the form of a loop. Figure 8.2 illustrated this in terms of the budget setting process; Figure 13.1 presents the same loop in the wider context of performance reporting in general.

From Figure 13.1, it is clear that reporting outcomes, and their subsequent review, are essential parts of the feedback loop and hence an essential part of management. The information collected, reported and used to assist the management process at any and all stages in the loop is called 'management information'. This is a generic term which is self-defining – any facts or figures that are deemed necessary or useful to the management process automatically become 'management information'. Management information is not to be confused with raw data which needs to be processed before it can be used for decision-making purposes. For example, the record of a single payment transaction is of little use until it is aggregated with similar transactions and reported to the spending manager.

Given the importance of financial management in the NHS, the reporting of performance in both financial and other terms that may impact on finance cannot be considered an optional or incidental activity; it is an absolute and unavoidable necessity. There are three distinct but interrelated areas of performance that warrant particular consideration. These are:

- financial recording and reporting
- functional activity recording and reporting
- patient activity recording and reporting.

The next sections of this chapter discuss each of these in isolation, and then gives an overview in the form of an examination of the means and extent by which they are interrelated through case mix management systems.

The aims of this chapter are to:

- give an overview of the accounting system in practice;
- show how information is summarized and fed into the control system;
- explain the budget hierarchy;
- describe how case mix management is operated.

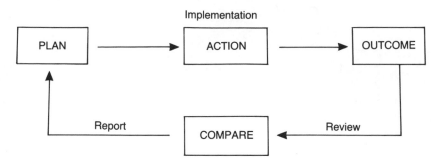

Figure 13.1 Management feedback loop.

Recording and reporting financial performance

DMUs and trusts spend many millions of pounds delivering health care each year, and it is essential that a full and accurate record is kept of how this money is spent. This is important for two purposes:

- **financial accounting**, so that proper books of account may be maintained;
- **management accounting**, so that performance against budgets and any other financial goals may be monitored.

The way in which information is to be reported determines the manner in which it is recorded. This is clear from an overview of the entire financial information recording and reporting process, starting at the individual transaction level and building up to the top-level budget reports. This process is illustrated in Figure 13.2.

The first principle of any accounting system is that every single financial transaction must be recorded at the earliest possible point. The manner in which the initial record is made must be able to support both statutory accounting and the management reporting requirements, and so, whatever financial coding structure is selected, it must provide the ability to report in many different ways. The first step of this process is to attach to each transaction a valid financial code to identify its nature. To be able to account, to the required level of detail, for the multitude of different transactions which may take place, a DMU/trust must have an extensive and well-defined financial coding structure. Combining the huge variety of different items with the wide range of reporting requirements means that tens or even hundreds of thousands of different financial codes are required.

The level at which financial transactions are coded should be, in theory, the lowest one at which financial reporting, whether statutory or for management purposes, is required. In practice, the ever-increasing demand for greater and greater cost detail at patient, procedure or DRG level means that this is not always possible within the ledger system, and some form of subsequent disaggregation of costs to the very lowest reporting level is normally unavoidable. Case mix management systems can be a useful tool in this area, and this topic is discussed towards the end of the chapter.

Handling the quantity of financial data generated can only be undertaken with the aid of computer-based accounting systems. To accommodate all the complexities, health authorities and trusts invest substantial sums of money in financial ledger systems. These are basically computerized 'books (or ledgers) of account', and provide

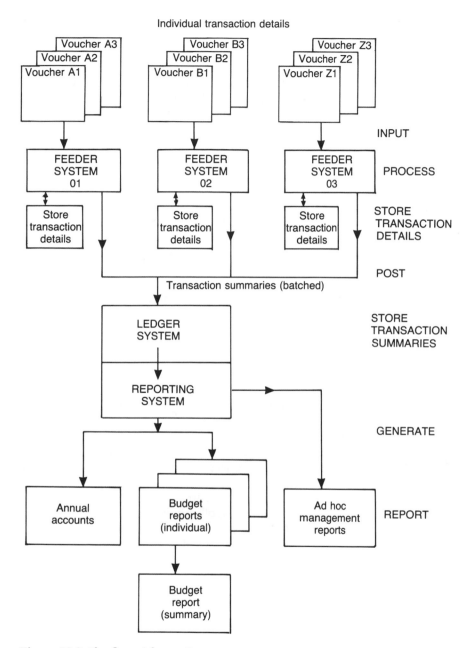

Figure 13.2 The financial reporting system.

the facility to allow financial transactions to be recorded using a predefined financial coding structure. Actual costs incurred and recorded in the ledger system can then be used both to produce the annual financial accounts and to match against the planned costs to determine the budget position. Some financial ledger systems provide their own reporting facilities for this, whilst with other systems such facilities are provided by a separate reporting system, but with electronic links between the two.

There are a wide selection of ledger and ledger/reporting systems in use in the NHS. These range from systems supplied by a number of commercial organizations to systems originally developed by Health Service regions such as the Interactive Resource Information System (IRIS). Traditionally they have been mainframe systems purchased or developed on a regional basis. The ever-increasing power of the minicomputer and the added needs imposed by the market environment has seen a break with tradition in recent years as trusts seek out systems that best meet their local needs.

At this point an important distinction must be made between the processing of transactions and the storing of the results. Whilst all costs are stored in the ledger against their respective financial codes, the actual processing of the tens or hundreds of thousands of individual transactions that give rise to these costs usually takes place outside of the ledger system in what are known as feeder systems. There are a number of these, each designed to process a particular type of transaction, of which the most common are:

- salaries and wages (weekly, monthly and urgent)
- travelling expenses
- creditor payments
- manual creditor payments
- stores – stock
- stores – non-stock
- debtors
- collection and deposit sheets
- journals
- capital charges
- certain departmental systems may also provide stock and non-stock control modules and thereby act as feeder systems to the ledger system.

Each different feeder system is purpose-designed to handle very specific types of transactions. For example, a payroll system processes salaries and wages for weekly and monthly paid staff and is capable of undertaking the various complex calculations involved with the payments due to the many professions and disciplines employed in the NHS. Quite often these feeder systems have been acquired over a period of time and may have been provided by a range of different suppliers, so there is unlikely to be much compatibility between their technical designs.

Due to the sheer volume of transactions involved in any one system it is quite normal for the feeder systems to pass across (or 'post') to the ledger system an aggregation or summarization of groups or 'batches' of transactions attributable to each financial code, rather than details of each individual transaction. Figure 13.3 illustrates this, and some of the following points. The batch used is either some obvious subdivision of a cyclical process – for example, a weekly or monthly payroll – or, for less cyclical transactions, a locally decided division is applied, for example every 50 bills raised.

The ledger system receives regular batch inputs from each feeder system, and each of these is recorded in a specific **ledger month**. As the name implies the ledger month is a simple division of the records stored in the ledger system into the time periods to which they relate. Normally there are twelve ledger months, being one for

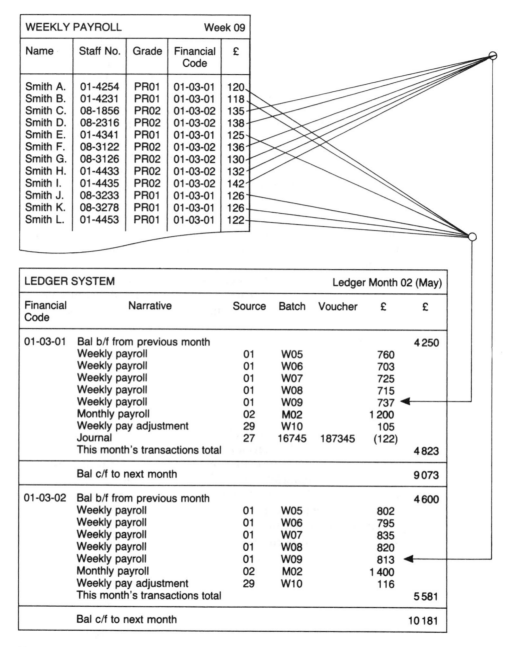

WEEKLY PAYROLL			Week 09	
Name	Staff No.	Grade	Financial Code	£
Smith A.	01-4254	PR01	01-03-01	120
Smith B.	01-4231	PR01	01-03-01	118
Smith C.	08-1856	PR02	01-03-02	135
Smith D.	08-2316	PR02	01-03-02	138
Smith E.	01-4341	PR01	01-03-01	125
Smith F.	08-3122	PR02	01-03-02	136
Smith G.	08-3126	PR02	01-03-02	130
Smith H.	01-4433	PR02	01-03-02	132
Smith I.	01-4435	PR02	01-03-02	142
Smith J.	08-3233	PR01	01-03-01	126
Smith K.	08-3278	PR01	01-03-01	126
Smith L.	01-4453	PR01	01-03-01	122

LEDGER SYSTEM					Ledger Month 02 (May)		
Financial Code	Narrative	Source	Batch	Voucher	£	£	
01-03-01	Bal b/f from previous month					4 250
	Weekly payroll	01	W05		760	
	Weekly payroll	01	W06		703	
	Weekly payroll	01	W07		725	
	Weekly payroll	01	W08		715	
	Weekly payroll	01	W09		737	
	Monthly payroll	02	M02		1 200	
	Weekly pay adjustment	29	W10		105	
	Journal	27	16745	187345	(122)	
	This month's transactions total					4 823
	Bal c/f to next month					9 073
01-03-02	Bal b/f from previous month					4 600
	Weekly payroll	01	W05		802	
	Weekly payroll	01	W06		795	
	Weekly payroll	01	W07		835	
	Weekly payroll	01	W08		820	
	Weekly payroll	01	W09		813	
	Monthly payroll	02	M02		1 400	
	Weekly pay adjustment	29	W10		116	
	This month's transactions total					5 581
	Bal c/f to next month					10 181

Notes: b/f = brought forward
c/f = carried forward

Figure 13.3 Links between feeder systems and the ledger system.

each calender month, plus a 'month 13' which is used to close down the accounts at the end of the financial year.

Certain cyclical transactions, such as weekly payroll and creditor payments, have to be batched on a weekly basis, and this causes the problem of matching 52 batches to twelve ledger months. A decision has to be made at the start of the year as to which weekly runs are to be fed into which ledger months. For example, it may be decided that Weeks 01 to 04 are to be fed into April (Month 01) and Weeks 05 to 09 fed into May (Month 02). To correct the fact that at the end of April there is a budget for one twelfth of the year, which is four and a bit weeks, but expenditure for only four weeks, an estimate of the 'missing' expenditure has to be made, and temporary month-end creditors posted in the ledger. Without these the staff budgets would not reflect the true financial position. Similarly it has to be ensured that all invoices for goods that have actually been received by the end of the month are included as temporary month-end creditors, even if they have not been paid. Month-end creditors are either calculated or estimated by the feeder systems or the ledger system itself, or have to be calculated manually and input as journal entries.

During the year it is inevitable that queries of one form or another arise in relation to the costs stored in the ledger system. Budget managers want detailed breakdowns of the costs for which they are responsible and which are charged to their budgets, even if only on an exception basis. Simply telling a budget manager that, for example, they spent £5581 on the weekly pay of a particular grade of staff last month is not satisfactory, especially if this is different from the budgeted cost. Budget managers need a much greater degree of detail and, because no more detail is stored in the ledger system, it can only be found by going back to the original feeder system.

In order to backtrack in this manner an **audit trail** is required. This trail can be picked up in the ledger system and identified first to the feeder system which created the batch, and to the unique number it allocated to the batch known as the batch identifier. In the example shown in Figure 13.3 the weekly payroll is identified by the 'Source' number = 01, and the week 09 pay is identified by the batch number = W09.

What may then be needed from the feeder system is a detailed breakdown of each of the financial code totals it has produced when creating the batch. In the example, such management information might take the form of a listing of all weekly paid staff sorted by financial code and sub-totalled each time the code changes to identify a change of sub-group. Analyses of this type are available to various degrees of comprehensiveness, depending upon the capability of the system.

Having examined this detail it may be wished to go back even further, perhaps first to obtain an even greater level of analysis. Continuing with the example, this might mean obtaining an analysis of overtime costs, sickness absence or bonus payments for each member of staff. The level to which such detail can be reported by a computer-based feeder system is determined by its design capability. Nearly all feeder systems more than a few years old were designed primarily for processing and not for reporting, with the result that finance departments still spend a lot of time manually extracting *ad hoc* information from the bulk paper or microfiche output of feeder systems or from basic on-screen enquiries.

The next stage requires an examination of one or more individual transactions in detail. The audit trail provides the ability to trace every transaction back through the feeder system to the documentation that originated it, whether an invoice, pay card or stores issue note. One more basic principle to be aware of is that a complete audit trail at all stages is a fundamental requirement if any sense is to be made of financial information batch-posted to the ledger and hence is a fundamental part of resource management.

Feeder systems contain all the basic information on the costs which result from resource consumption. However, reporting on resource consumption is not just a matter of reporting pounds and pence; it also involves providing management information on levels and types of consumption and then assigning a cost to these. The availability and suitability of such management information from feeder systems is crucial to proper resource management and hence to financial management. One major way of improving financial management is to ensure such availability, perhaps even more so than in trying to develop hugely complex budget reporting mechanisms.

Rather than await the month-end budget reports to determine the financial position, the extraction of suitable management information from feeder systems as soon as each batch has been processed provides a highly valuable tool. This may not be technically possible every week, but, as a minimum, there should be the aim of producing such management information in respect of the major feeder systems for all batches in a month immediately after the close of the final day of the month. This approach is useful because there can be a gap of six or seven weeks between the processing of some transactions and their inclusion in the budget reports. To be of most use, information should be acted on as soon as possible, and the elimination of delays by issuing summary information as soon as it is available enables management to respond more promptly.

Reports are only as accurate as far as the detailed supporting information is itself accurate. If costs are missing from the ledger or are incorrectly coded this inevitably reduces the value of a report. Where this becomes a frequent occurrence it reduces user trust, and may even destroy the credibility of all information produced by the financial systems. Users may even develop alternative systems of their own, thereby duplicating effort.

Costs which are missing from the ledger arise because they have not been captured by the feeder systems. A system that ensures the thorough calculation of the temporary month-end creditors and inclusion of these in the ledger via journal entries should serve to address this potential problem. The problem of incorrect coding can be more difficult to control, especially if there are several stages in the process by which transactions are initiated. There are three types of 'incorrect' code:

- missing codes, i.e. transactions that have been processed without any code being attached;
- invalid codes, i.e. codes that do not exist in the financial coding structure;
- valid codes, i.e. codes that do exist, but that are incorrect for the particular transaction.

In the first two cases such problems may be discovered when the transaction is input to the feeder system, but only where the feeder systems have the capability of accessing a list of valid codes or highlighting missing codes. More commonly the error is picked up at the ledger posting stage and all transactions with missing or invalid codes are then posted to an account called **error suspense**. Each of these has to be examined, another important function of the audit trail, and corrected so that the error suspense account can be 'cleared'. The third type of error is more difficult to detect. Most frequently it is discovered when budget managers query unexpected figures on their budget reports. This is corrected by re-coding to the correct code, but the effect of the correction does not appear in the reports until they are next issued.

These problems can be avoided if everything is correctly coded first time. The best way of ensuring this is by implementing a system of **source coding**, whereby all transactions are coded at the stage of initiation, i.e. at their source, and the onus is placed firmly upon those having managerial responsibility for the financial consequences. Suitable training is required, both as to the structure of the coding system and the importance of correct coding.

Integrated feeder systems

Some of the more modern ledger systems have the capability to examine individual transactions in a feeder system directly by electronic communication. With others such examination may only be possible by leaving the ledger system and directly accessing the feeder system. The former capability is variously described as 'integrated' or 'interactive' enquiry, whilst the latter is known by a number of terms, including 'remote' enquiry. Truly integrated financial systems are still very much in their infancy in the NHS, but their major advantage lies in the ready access they provide from the ledger to supporting transaction details. This contrasts with the laborious and time-consuming added steps that are involved in constantly having to access the ledger and remote feeder systems in turn as queries are investigated. Where feeder systems are not truly integrated there is sometimes the capability of feeding across to the ledger for storage selected data items for each transaction. Such detail may be held in the ledger for a fairly short period, perhaps just a month or a few months, whilst queries are resolved.

Batch input systems

For any batch system, the update timetable must be known if any sense is to be made of the information recorded in the ledger. For example, the daily stores stock issues are processed by the feeder system as they are made. If the batch update of the ledger is made at the end of each week, then a comparison made part way through a week between the issues for the year shown in the feeder system and the total shown in the ledger will disclose a discrepancy equal to the issues chargeable to that code for the week to date. One of the other problems with remote systems is reconciling total amounts stored in the ledger to the detailed figures stored in the feeder system. Whilst these should tie up exactly it depends on how well the management information extraction routines have been written.

Budget performance reporting

Having established the means by which financial data is recorded in the ledger system the next consideration is how it is reported in terms of budget performance. Basic budget setting principles include identifying, within the management hierarchy, a manager responsible for the performance of each budget. Such managers require regular progress reports, to enable them to monitor actual resource consumption against the planned level. Normally this takes the form of each manager receiving one or more monthly detailed **budget reports**.

The number and format of these reports varies considerably between DMUs/trusts, but generally each one relates to a group of interdependent or similar expenditure types, with each individual budget amount identified on a separate 'line' of the report. For example, a clinical directorate may have individual nursing budgets for each of its wards, and the report may be designed to provide a different line for each grade of nursing staff.

Performance evaluation is always best undertaken on a one-to-one matching of budget and actual, and so the budget manager requires actual budget performance figures to the same level of detail as that at which the budgets were set, i.e. on a line-by-line basis. This is achieved by aggregating for each report line the financial codes against which the actual level of matching expenditure has been coded and then adjusting for any apportionments and recharges as necessary. The specific means by which this is undertaken depends upon the coding structure and the ledger/reporting system being used. There is little to be gained by setting budgets at a level of detail below which actual performance can accurately be reported.

Budget performance may also be reported using measures of consumption other than finance. Commonly, staff budgets also indicate the number of whole time equivalent (WTE) staff numbers employed in the period for comparison to budgeted WTE amounts. Non-staff budgets may also provide an indication of activity levels for comparison with budgeted activity levels, and this is discussed in the next section in this chapter.

Budgeted and actual performance figures are normally presented for the current reporting month ('current' amounts) and for the entire year to date ('cumulative' amounts). This assists in the identification of trends, which are far more indicative of actual or potential problems and of the likely year-end position than any single month's performance.

The financial reporting mechanism provides a means whereby the performance of several different low-level budget reports are summarized. Managers at increasingly higher levels within the reporting hierarchy require less and less detail and are increasingly interested in the overall position of their area of responsibility. At the highest level, the board of directors needs an accurate statement of budget position for the entire DMU/trust. The basic principle of any budget reporting structure is that it should reflect the management reporting hierarchy, and a typical budget report summarization method is illustrated in Figure 13.4.

Inevitably, queries are raised at all levels and, once again, an audit trail must be present to allow the tracing of amounts shown on summary and detailed reports back to financial codes. Another important principle connected with this is that there must be controls built into the budget reporting system to ensure that the total income and expenditure amounts recorded in the ledger system exactly equals the sum of the detailed budget reports and that, in turn, must exactly equal the sum of the summary budget reports. If this is not the case, it means that either some income or expenditure has been totally missed from the reports, or that some has been reported upon twice. In either case a false position is presented.

Ad hoc reports may be requested to assist in the overall financial management process. Depending upon their content and complexity it may be possible to produce these using report generation facilities built in to the reporting system, or they may have to be manually extracted from the ledger.

The presentation of purely financial information generally is not enough to assess overall performance. It has to be linked to functional and patient activity levels if any real understanding of the facts behind the figures is to be gained. The following two sections consider the recording and reporting of such information.

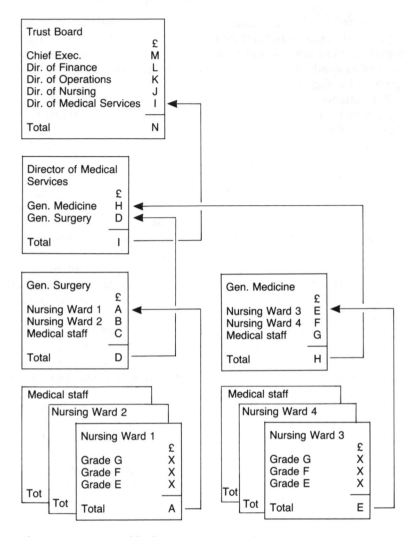

Figure 13.4 A typical budget summarization hierarchy.

Recording and reporting functional activity performance

Each of the different functional departments exists to provide a particular service or group of services. Costs are incurred as a result of this provision, some of which are 'fixed' by nature and some of which are 'variable'. Identification of costs and how they are expected to behave enables a budget, based on the planned level of activity, to be prepared for each function. Actual performance is then compared with the expected outcome by the use of variance analysis, and this comparison can only take place if both accurate and appropriate financial data and activity data are available.

Financial recording and reporting systems, as discussed in the previous section, have been in use in the NHS for decades. Their functionality, although often very basic compared to those of commercial organizations, is well tried and tested and their strengths and weaknesses known. In contrast, functional activity and workload recording and reporting systems do not, in general, have such a lengthy history of development or widespread use. Their background often lies in the adaptation or extension of existing systems, both computer-based and manual, designed for the operational purpose of running or managing a department. The way in which such a system operates is now considered in the context of the pharmacy department.

A computer-based pharmacy stock-control system can be used to keep a record of drugs received from suppliers and of drugs issued, on a drug-by-drug basis. At this level this should be a straightforward task, and basic stock-control systems which can handle this work have been available for many years. Each individual transaction has to be recorded and, at a minimum, must identify the drug and the quantity being received or issued. It is then a simple matter for the system to highlight those drugs for which stock levels are falling below a pre-set level.

Additional management information on resource consumption becomes available if the minimum recording requirement for transactions on the issues side is increased to identify, as a matter of routine, some additional feature, such as the prescribing doctor or the specialty or the ward or even the patient. Introducing such a change requires a great deal of development of both the computer system and, even more importantly, the system by which these new basic details are identified to the pharmacy.

The required changes in the use of the system can be investigated by assuming as an example that a trust has decided that each clinical directorate should become responsible for a number of non-staff budgets, including drugs. The setting of an individual drugs budget for each directorate is relatively simple. Even without computer systems the once-a-year exercise can be undertaken manually using historical data adjusted as appropriate. It is more difficult to ensure that the system by which actual drug usage is recorded is sufficiently robust to allow the accurate identification of drug issues, and their associated cost, to directorates each month. A major responsibility lies with all prescribing clinicians to ensure that prescription scripts accurately identify the directorate which is to bear the cost. If directorates share a ward and there is a common drug stock at ward level then the system must allow the analysis of ward drug usage between directorates. At the pharmacy end, the principal pharmacist must ensure that the pharmacy staff correctly use the recording system and that all errors are 'trapped' prior to entry.

The total cost of drugs is normally charged in the ledger to the pharmacy at the time of purchase. The cost of subsequent issues is then recharged in the ledger to directorates, either directly through electronic links or by the raising of journal entries. The pharmacy system must itself be capable of producing a detailed breakdown of the cost of these issues in a format which is suitable for monitoring purposes and which maintains a verifiable audit trail.

Similar comments can be made in terms of other functional areas where management information systems often started life as operational tools, perhaps for booking patients or recording test results, or generally may originally have performed simple administrative tasks. In all of these cases the same basic principles apply to activity recording systems as to financial systems: the information extracted is only as good as the data fed in, and this is only as good as the systems that capture and process the data for input. One of the dangers to be avoided when developing activity or workload recording systems, whether computer-based or manual, is in concentrating on the process only from the **data input** stage onwards with little consideration of the earlier **data capture** steps.

Recording and reporting patient activity

Ultimately, all services are provided as part of the overall delivery of health care to patients. Budget setting is undertaken on the basis of functional and departmental activity levels which are in turn intended to be directly related to planned patient activity. Under the contracting arrangements a provider's funding is obtained almost entirely through the fulfilment of patient contracts, which are themselves expressions of planned patient activity. Accurate and detailed recording and reporting of patient activity is essential as it is strongly linked with the income and expenditure budgets.

Unlike financial systems, which have always been an absolute and unavoidable requirement, patient administration systems in the past have not been essential to financial management and have not always been seen as worthy of substantial investment. However, various systems did exist even prior to contracting, and recording patient activity in the hospital sector is undertaken by what are generically termed 'patient administration' or 'patient management' systems. As with functional systems, these come in a number of guises, both computer-based and manual, and often a combination of both. For many years they were designed to cope primarily with the operational requirements of simple patient record-keeping and little, if any, management information was sought from them. Despite initiatives such as resource management, which placed an increased importance upon their management information capabilities, most computer-based patient administration systems were, until recently, surprisingly poorly developed when compared with other systems, although there were exceptions. This situation arose because of a number of factors, not least of which is the huge development costs of producing such a system.

The introduction of contracting arrangements brought about dramatic changes in the need for patient activity data. Under the new regime a provider has to be able to identify, for each and every patient:

- a purchaser, including GP fundholders, as it is from these that payment of the treatment is received;
- a contract, as this sets out the terms of payment;
- the correct 'currency' or unit of contract, e.g. in-patient days, deaths and discharges.

The correct identification of patients chargeable under the extra contractual referral arrangements is of particular importance, and it must be done within the correct timescale. All of these requirements must be met by the provision of minimum data sets for each patient. As a result, in a relatively short timescale, patient administration systems were suddenly expected to be able to record, process and report this huge additional amount of detail.

The new requirements have been met in a number of ways, and to varying degrees of satisfaction. None of the then existing computer-based systems were able comprehensively to provide all of the facilities needed under the contracting arrangements, largely because they had never been designed for such a role. Over a period of time, many have been further developed to cope with the new recording requirements with varying degrees of success. Various approaches have also been adopted on the reporting side. In some cases the patient administration systems have themselves been developed in this area, whilst in others an interface with other software products providing suitable reporting capabilities has been attempted. In yet other cases totally new reporting products have been specifically designed and developed. The 'CoManDS' (Contract Management and Decision Support) system, developed by the South Glamorgan Health Authority and jointly funded with the Welsh Office, is perhaps the most ambitious and successful of these, using powerful microcomputer hardware and software to provide highly sophisticated and flexible reporting tools in respect of raw patient data downloaded from a mainframe patient administration system.

The picture is different in the community sector where a much higher proportion of 'functional' activity can be related directly to individual patients. The recent development work that has taken place recognizes the operational difficulties of data collection and concentrated on the provision of computer-based systems capable of recording patient-based activity details via hand-held or lap-top computers, using direct keyboard entry or bar codes. Once again the emphasis has been on operational requirements and the collection of summary information for statutory or regulatory returns, with general management information on performance being a closely following secondary interest.

For contracting purposes the detail provided by the new systems may be far more than is required, particularly where block contracts have been agreed. Some community services providers have postponed making substantial investments in patient-based systems and have opted to remain with or to acquire simpler and cheaper employee-based paper-driven systems to meet their short- to medium-term needs. An example of such a package is 'CHAAP' (Community Health Activity Analysis Package), a purpose-built microcomputer system in use in the South Glamorgan Health Authority Community Services Unit.

All of the above recognizes the importance of accurate patient activity recording and reporting in terms of financial management, and the same basic principles as for financial and functional activity performance apply. In particular, a discipline similar to that suggested for accurate financial coding needs to be applied when coding patients in any way. Responsibility for the final identification of a patient to a contract should lie with those best placed to determine this and whose finances such identification most directly affect, namely the clinical managers of contracts.

In conclusion, the introduction of the contracting regime has forced major developments and improvements in patient activity recording and reporting on a wide scale. Given the direct link between resource consumption and patient activity an outside observer might assume that the consideration of these two factors in the light of each other would long have been a basic requirement. Much, but not all, of the fault for the previous lack of development lies with the basic overall NHS funding allocation method in use in the pre-contracting period which did not match funding to patient activity, and so provided little incentive to use limited funds to develop such systems.

Case mix management systems

One development which did provide some incentive was the introduction of the Resource Management Initiative (RMI) and the development of the case mix manage-

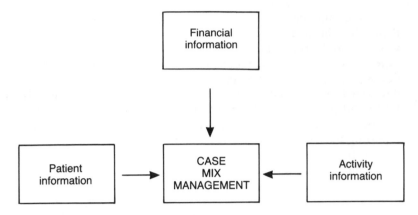

Figure 13.5 A basic case mix management system.

ment systems. The RMI has already been discussed, and this section now briefly considers case mix management in the context of performance recording and reporting. Case mix is a powerful means of linking financial and non-financial information in a manner meaningful to managers and clinicians alike. It provides a management tool for planning and budgeting for clinical activity and, properly constructed, can form the basis of a clinical audit.

Case mix management is an approach to resource management that involves the matching of patient-related activity or workload information with associated patient resource consumption information in the form of financial data. This is achieved by recording, for each individual patient, the details of all 'interventions' and 'events' which take place as part of the provision of health care. The volume of data involved requires case mix management to be a computer-based system, and it usually involves the integration of financial and non-financial 'feeder' systems which pass data to a case mix system. This is illustrated in an over-simplified way in Figure 13.5.

Each intervention or event is chargeable at a standard, or average, cost derived from standard protocols of care, determined and agreed by clinical staff. The case mix system then monitors patients against these protocols.

Information is collated for groupings of patients to provide actual average costs, which are compared with the predetermined target standard costs for that grouping . This grouping approach is required because of the impossibility of identifying all actual costs directly to individual patients. Patients must be grouped in a clinically meaningful way. This demands a standard and reliable method of classification which is usually provided by the use of diagnosis related groupings (DRGs).

In the contracting environment a case mix system becomes the primary source of information for the contract pricing mechanism and an essential prerequisite to the derivation of meaningful contract prices below the broad specialty level. The importance of this development both now and in the future cannot be under-estimated, and as to the question of whether a provider can afford to make the substantial investment required, it is more a matter of whether it can afford not to.

Conclusion

Non-financial information systems in the NHS have developed in a fragmented way on an *ad hoc* basis to meet specific, often localized, requirements. The introduction of contracting has stimulated the creation of systems which produce reports incorporating many types of data, such as that measured in financial terms or that relating to patients. The foundation of these systems is to ensure that the initial record is created with the amount of detail needed to produce a report dealing with the most specific material. Above that level, reports of decreasing complexity and increasing generality can be created by aggregation. In this way, the degree of detail in each report can be matched to the amount required by the recipient.

Questions

1. Financial management, like any form of management, is a continuous process. Why must this be so?
2. How are the three key facets of performance – finance, functional activity and patient activity levels – brought together, and why is this so important?
3. The manner by which and level of detail at which transactions are stored is determined by what? What are the basic principles of reporting such detail?
4. Accurate identification of all types of transactions via a predefined coding structure is important. Why is this? Explain and illustrate with an example how a system to ensure accurate coding can be introduced for any one transaction/activity flow in each of the areas of:

   - financial coding (for example payroll, non-staff ordering);
   - recording and apportionment of functional activity (for example radiology, pharmacy, pathology);
   - recording patient activity for matching against contracts.

5. 'The budget reporting structure should reflect the management reporting structure.' What problems would be caused if this were not so? How many levels of budget summarization are required within a reporting hierarchy, and how is this determined?
6. How are financial reports and clinical activity interlinked? Is it possible to have one without the other?
7. Coding transactions is used more for management information requirements than to fulfil statutory reporting needs, therefore managers have a vested interest in ensuring that coding is performed accurately and promptly. Why does coding carry such low esteem in any organization when it is so inherently important?
8. What are the main advantages and disadvanges of integrated and batch feeder systems? Which system best suits the needs of a large NHS trust?
9. 'To establish a budget is relatively easy; it is in the recording of performance where the difficulties lie.' Discuss.

14

Financial regulation in NHS trusts

AIMS

Financial management is a process which requires regulation by feedback and response so that any divergence from planned results can be measured and adjusted for. The purpose of a regulatory mechanism is to ensure that the feedback is **automatically** communicated to those in the appropriate position to take any action that is within their authority to ensure that the goals are achieved.

The ultimate responsibility for financial management within an NHS trust lies with the trust board of directors. They must ensure that suitable regulatory mechanisms are in place within the trust and that the responsibility entrusted to each employee is properly fulfilled. However, the board is itself answerable to a higher authority, which for the purposes of this chapter we shall call 'the centre'. That higher authority has its own responsibilities and so, by the same token, a board's actions must be subject to some form of regulation and must be bounded within clearly established parameters.

There is a wide range of regulatory mechanisms in place, and the aims of this chapter are to:

- outline the composition and duties of the trust board of directors;
- show how regulation of the financial aspects of the trust is achieved through structure, procedure, planning, accountability and financing;
- map the limits of the freedom of action within which trusts have to operate.

Regulation through structure and procedure

All trusts are free to exercise, within the prescribed limits, the powers given to them by the NHS and Community Care Act 1990. The powers and authority of an individual trust are limited because each one is established to perform a particular function or set of functions, and it can only operate in such a way as to fulfil these

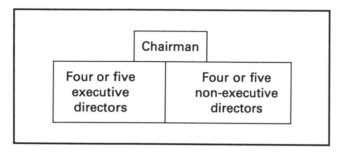

Figure 14.1 Composition of an NHS trust board of directors.

functions. Each trust is run by a board of directors, the composition of which is outlined in Figure 14.1.

The board has a maximum of eleven members, including the chairman, and a minimum of nine. The directors are all full and equal members of the board, and are appointed as follows:

- a non-executive chairman, who is appointed by the Secretary of State;
- a maximum of five executive directors which must include a:
  - chief executive
  - director of finance
  - medical director or equivalent
  - nursing director or equivalent;
- an equal number of non-executive directors. One of these must be a representative of the relevant university if a trust has a significant commitment to undergraduate medical teaching. The non-executive directors are not chosen as representatives of any particular interest group. Their selection is based on the personal contribution they can make to the management of the trust, which may stem from the experience or expertise they have in areas such as law, commerce, banking, finance, education and general service to the community.

Once appointed, the board has to attend to its three key areas of corporate responsibility, which are to:

- determine and agree the overall strategic policies of the trust;
- monitor the execution of these policies;
- ensure the ongoing financial viability of the trust.

The last of these, ensuring financial viability, leads to the detailed financial responsibilities of the trust board of which there are two main ones and two supplementary ones:

- Main financial responsibilities:
  - The trust must break even on its income and expenditure account, after payment of interest and dividends, taking one year with another.
  - The trust must make the required rate of return on its net assets, which is expressed as its financial target.
  - The trust must operate within its external financing limit which is set centrally each year.
- Supplementary financial responsibilities:

– A sound system of financial management must be in place.
– Appropriate standing financial instructions must be adopted and complied with.

Turning to the individual board members, the chief executive is appointed by the chairman and non-executive directors and has executive responsibility for the performance of all of the trust functions including:

- implementation and achievement of the trust policies;
- ensuring the financial viability of the trust and the meeting of its financial obligations;
- day-to-day management of the trust's affairs.

The other executive directors are appointed by the chairman, non-executive directors and chief executive and they too have particular responsibilities. Those of the director of finance can include ensuring that:

- the financial policies of the trust are implemented;
- proper systems of financial management and control are in place and maintained;
- adequate financial records are maintained of the trust's business affairs;
- appropriate financial advice is provided to the chief executive and to the board to allow them to discharge their duties.

Whilst the chief executive has overall executive responsibility for the performance of the trust, other directors have responsibility for specific areas. For example, the medical and nursing directors provide professional advice and guidance on the practical implications of the trust's policies on patients and patient care. The director of finance has a duty to provide appropriate and adequate financial advice both to the board and the chief executive. This requires the existence, maintenance and operation of systems of financial control and accounting, for which the finance director is also responsible.

Trusts are free to develop any management structures and hierarchies beneath board level that they determine best suits their particular local needs. This structure must be clearly defined, and must reflect the responsibilities of the board members themselves. The chief executive and director of finance are authorized to delegate certain responsibilities to nominated officers, although the trust board is expected to review the appropriateness of this delegation at regular intervals. Indeed the purpose of a management hierarchy is to ensure that decision-making is delegated to an appropriate level. However, it is important that at all times the decision-making process is regulated so as to remain within the limitations of the trust's approved functions and to ensure that its declared and agreed policies are achieved in the way intended.

Given the importance that all of the trust's activities are properly regulated, documentation is required to convey to managers the limits of their power and authority and the manner in which the business of the trust is to be conducted. This regulatory documentation must be comprehensive where financial matters are concerned, and the way in which this basic requirement is fulfilled is in the form of a hierarchy, as illustrated in Figure 14.2.

The elements shown in Figure 14.2, which all contribute to control through procedure, are now considered in turn:

- **Standing Orders** are formulated and agreed by the trust board and set out the general terms by which the business of the board and of the trust is conducted.

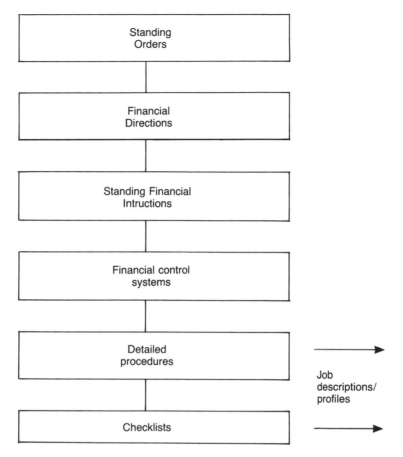

Figure 14.2 The hierarchy of control.

These are considered to be the ultimate governing principles of the activities of the trust and each of its directors and employees.

- **Financial Directions** are formulated by the director of finance and agreed by the trust board. They set out particular major responsibilities of the director of finance and 'direct' the undertaking of certain duties. They also place certain key responsibilities upon other board members, particularly the chief executive.
- **Standing Financial Instructions (SFIs)** are also formulated by the director of finance and agreed by the trust board. They set out the manner in which the requirements of the Standing Orders and Financial Directions are to be applied, and it is mandatory for all employees to follow them. Their purpose has been defined as follows:

  > Standing Financial Instructions are issued for the regulation of the conduct of the Trust, its Directors, Officers and Agents in relation to all financial matters. They shall have effect as if incorporated in the Standing Orders of the Trust.
  >
  > NHS Trusts Finance Manual.

These provide more detailed guidance of the roles and responsibilities of the board

and its members from a financial perspective. They are expected as a minimum to regulate conduct in the following financial areas:
- business plans and estimates
- contracting
- budgets
- income
- annual accounts and reports
- bank accounts
- investments
- external borrowing and originating debt
- security of assets
- payment of staff
- payment of accounts
- purchasing
- stores
- patients' property
- data processing
- internal audit
- non-exchequer funds.

The SFIs do not provide the detailed technical method by which financial regulation is achieved. Rather, they identify the overall means by specifying particular responsibilities arising in the main areas listed above. A further essential feature is to stipulate financial limits for different transaction types above which higher authority must be sought to proceed. The SFIs require review from time to time to ensure that currently they meet the requirements of the trust and are amended to suit locally changing circumstances.

- **Financial control systems (FCS)** have to be complied with by all employees and are recorded in a substantial document which sets out in detail the main systems in place to ensure financial control and the proper safeguarding of the trust assets and resources. The financial control systems are concerned with complete processes and document each step of each of the financial systems necessary for the running of a trust, clearly identifying:
  - the flow of responsibility at each stage in the process
  - the flow of documentation and information
  - the safeguards built in to ensure internal control, separation of duties and internal checking.

For example, the financial control system which deals with the ordering, receiving and paying for goods or services demonstrates the separation of duties between the individual responsible for raising the order, the individual responsible for receiving the goods, and the individual responsible for authorizing payment against the order and the goods-received notification.

- **Procedures** are recorded in detail for each of the major steps within the financial control system. These are designed either to set out the steps to be followed for each postholder involved in the process (post-oriented), or the steps followed within a department (function-oriented). For any financial control system there are a number of written procedures, some following on in sequence, with others running in parallel. Thus the individual responsible for ordering goods and services has a written procedure to follow which sets out the method for ordering goods and services and the limits of authority in different circumstances.

A number of additional written procedures have to be developed for complementary and supporting activities which do not directly impact on the financial performance or the financial control within a trust. For example, systems are required to deal with health and safety at work, disciplinary matters and enrolment of staff. All such procedures are beneficial in assisting to identify clearly a postholder's role, power and authority.

- **Checklists** are common within the finance discipline for each of the various stages within a particular procedure. These set out each of the tasks to be performed in their logical sequence so that the individual responsible for performing those tasks can then 'check off' each stage as it is completed. Checklists are particularly useful where relatively complex tasks have to be undertaken on a regular basis and are of great assistance where a task has to be undertaken by someone not familiar with it, perhaps through covering for absence or through taking up a new post.
- **Job descriptions/profiles** are not directly linked with the hierarchy outlined above, but the key tasks and roles undertaken by a postholder are to some extent reflected in their job description/profile.

Moving down through the various levels of documentation, there is an increasing detail of definition of responsibility. This reflects the fact that, at the top level, the strategic and policy decisions taken by senior managers and directors have to be translated into day-to-day operational activities, many of which are undertaken by junior staff. Without this regulatory mechanism providing clear direction there is no means to ensure compliance with declared policies and aims. Thus the conversion of strategic intent into detailed operational practices, supported by detailed documentation, is a key regulatory mechanism within the trust.

Regulation through planning

The short- and medium-term business intentions of the trust are expressed in the business plan. This reconciles with both the strategic planning intentions and the short-term operational plans and must also accord with centrally issued guidance. The business plan integrates with the financial proformas completed by the director of finance for submission both to the board and to the centre. Both of these must reconcile with the capital investment programme.

The financial proformas are an important tool for assessing and demonstrating the ongoing financial viability of the trust. Prior to any approval of trust status the proformas are completed by the applicant and are subject to vigorous scrutiny. Even after approval these proformas must be updated regularly and must be capable of direct reconciliation with the business planning process.

Many of the proformas are completed for a six-year period, which comprises the two prior years, the current year, and three future years. Taken together, these tables present the financial plans of the trust, allow an assessment of ongoing financial viability, and, once agreed with the centre, identify the permitted level of capital spend. The substance and purpose of each of the main tables in the set of proformas, which are described below, remain the same, although developments regularly take place in their detail. The main financial and related statements in the proformas are:

- **Income and expenditure accounts** which set out the projected income and expenditure, including interest and dividends payable by the trust, identifying the annual surplus or deficit. It shows in percentage terms the financial target performance, which is measured by the rate of return on net assets.

- **Balance sheets** to identify the fixed and current assets, current liabilities and capital debt of the trust. The capital debt is split between public dividend capital and interest bearing debt. There are other balancing reserve accounts for items such as revaluation of assets, donations and the accumulated balance on the income and expenditure account.
- **Source and application of funds statements** identify the anticipated source of funding that is available to the trust during the year and the intended application of it, with the overall net difference being the external financing requirement, which has to be funded by the **external financing limit** (EFL). The EFL is the net additional external financing that the trust is allowed to obtain, and is the difference between agreed total capital spending and the funding generated internally through such items as depreciation, land sales and surpluses on the income and expenditure account.
- **The statement of key assumptions** sets out the assumptions in the key areas of inflation, interest rates, level of capital debt and any growth over gross domestic product. These key assumptions play a vital role in determining the financial viability of the trust.
- **An analysis of income activity** to detail income over the main contract types, such as in-patients, out-patients and day cases, and by customer base, that is by purchaser. It also provides patient activity levels in actual terms for previous years and projected terms for current and future years. Ratios are calculated and included to demonstrate any change in efficiency over the period. The inclusion of details about patient activity levels is particularly important and they are a key variable in the costing/budgeting/pricing process.
- **Tangible fixed assets** are listed to support the calculation of fixed assets within the balance sheet, analysing them between: land; buildings, installations and fittings; and plant and equipment. The depreciation charges are included in this table, and the total to date deducted from the values of fixed assets to give their net current value, after depreciation. A second statement is completed in respect of any donated assets which are held.
- **Capital expenditure plans** are summarized for the trust for the current year and three future years. Schemes are identified by expenditure type and by major category. It is the capital investment plans and proposals that form the foundation of the trust's financial plans.
- **A capital scheme analysis** is completed for each project costing over a certain limit to provide further analysis and an explanation of the project.
- **The cash flow forecast (annual)** provides a projection of the monthly cash flow forecast and cash balance for the trust for the coming year of operation. It identifies any temporary borrowing requirement on a monthly basis.

It is the responsibility of the trust board, and the chief executive and director of finance, to monitor performance against the financial plans set out in the proformas. The formulating of these plans by the trust board, their subsequent agreement or otherwise by the centre, and the monitoring of achievement against plans all act as a regulatory mechanism.

Whilst the financial proformas summarize the financial plans of the trust for the current year and coming three years, it is the financial budgets developed within the trust that set out these plans in detail for the current year and for the coming year.

Specific responsibility is placed upon budget managers to maintain resource consumption within planned levels whilst at the same time achieving defined levels of activity or output. The delegation of responsibility is reflected in the delegation of these budgets. Operationally, budgets are a key regulatory mechanism. That is why an understanding of their purpose and a comprehension of their management and control is a key element in the achievement of the trust's overall policies and goals.

Regulation through accountability

The trust is externally accountable for its performance against its plans. Individual directors and managers, and all those with other delegated responsibility, are internally accountable to the chief executive and to the trust board for their own individual performance. This internal and external accountability are two further important manifestations of the regulatory mechanism, and are now each considered in more detail.

Internal accountability

Budgets provide a regulatory mechanism, and performance against them must be monitored and reported through the budget management hierarchy to the trust board. In terms of wider financial performance, there is internal accountability at all levels in the hierarchy and the main elements reported up to the board on a regular basis are as follows:

- income performance against target
- expenditure performance against target
- balance sheet
- cash flow position
- achievement against financial target (rate of return)
- take up of reserves, analysed by type of reserve.

Resource consumption is the key to financial performance, and so those responsible for initiating consumption must be accountable for it. Internal accountability arrangements must ensure the monitoring of both staff and non-staff resources in addition to the related expenditure. Actual income and expenditure are linked to activity levels and the internal accountability arrangements ensure the monitoring and reporting of activity against the planned levels determined by the contracts held. Although not directly a financial issue, the quality of delivery of service should also be subject to internal accountability as failure to meet agreed quality standards can have financial consequences in the medium or even the short term.

The internal audit service supports accountability. It has the responsibility and authority to examine, report upon and make recommendations in respect of any matter which could directly or indirectly affect the finances of the trust. These matters include, as a minimum, establishing or verifying the following:

- the relevance and suitability of established procedures, plans and policies and the extent of compliance;

- that adequate financial and related management controls are in place and are being complied with;
- the safeguarding of assets and interests from loss arising from fraud, theft, malpractice, waste, inefficient administration, poor value for money, extravagance and incompetence;
- efficient resource utilization;
- the accuracy, reliability and suitability of financial and non-financial management information and data.

External accountability

As part of the planning process, the trust prepares an annual business plan and an accompanying set of financial proformas. These are concerned not only with the past, current or projected performance and position in financial terms, but also in business and activity terms. Taken together, the financial and other data form part of the external regulatory mechanism. The plans are submitted to the centre for examination, and, once they have been approved, the trust is then accountable for actual performance against them. To ensure that the centre can perform its control function it requires regular resubmission of the financial proformas and the submission, to a specific timetable, of a number of different returns and statements. In addition, the centre requires details of high level performance indicators. The areas covered by the high level indicators and some examples of how measurement is carried out are as follows:

- **Activity levels** are reported in terms of verifiable facts such as the number of in-patient discharges, the number of day cases, and the total accident and emergency attendances.
- **Value for money** is measured by the bed occupancy rate, average length of stay, and theatre utilization.
- **Quality** encompasses a number of indicators such as waiting times for out-patient appointments and the number of cancelled planned out-patient sessions.
- **Financial management** reports summarize totals for such features as the net working balances and the cumulative surplus or deficit of payments against receipts.

In all of the above categories, the planned and actual figures are reported, and the variance between them shown. The results are then cross-referenced to exception reports to explain outcomes which differ from those predicted.

Accounting ratio analysis, as described in Chapter 5, is a popular and developing means of indicating any salient trends of a trust's financial performance during the year. This acts as an early warning mechanism to allow corrective action where financial difficulties are predicted.

At the end of each year a trust prepares and submits its annual statement of accounts, as a requirement imposed by statute. These are often referred to as the 'Körner accounts' and serve to demonstrate that a proper record of accounts has been maintained during the year. They also provide information on costs associated with defined workload activity on a functional basis to allow the derivation of costs per (Körner) unit of activity. The annual accounts of the trust are subject to an external audit each year, and, from time to time, the Audit Commission undertakes investigations, particularly on the value for money side aimed at assessing the efficiency and effectiveness of service delivery.

Regulation through financing

The three key financial responsibilities of the trust board are:

- to break even in terms of income and expenditure, taking one year on another;
- to achieve the target rate of return on net capital assets;
- to live within the external financing limit.

These primary parameters are used to regulate the financing of trusts. Within this framework there are at least two very useful means that can be used to fine-tune the regulatory mechanism:

- **External financing limit.** Each trust has a centrally approved annual capital spending limit set each year. The external financing limit effectively sets the limit on net borrowing that can be undertaken to finance the approved capital investment. This controls the overall change in levels of investment within a trust, that is the amount of public expenditure that a trust can undertake. An EFL can be positive, negative or neutral. The centre is able, by controlling the EFL of each individual trust, to ensure that the aggregate capital expenditure made available by the government is not exceeded.

  An EFL is **positive** where the trust's approved capital requirements exceed internally generated funds in the form of depreciation, revenue surpluses and changes in working capital balances. This allows the trust to borrow, or to reduce its investments, in order to finance the capital spending and effectively places a maximum limit on net borrowing.

  An EFL is **negative** where internally generated resources are greater than the approved capital requirements. The trust then uses these surplus funds to repay loans or can invest them for use in future years. A negative EFL in effect imposes a minimum net saving requirement.

  A **neutral** EFL occurs where the internally generated resources exactly match the approved capital requirements.

- **Dividend payable on public dividend capital.** In the medium term a dividend equivalent to the rate of interest on interest bearing debt is payable on public dividend capital. In the shorter term a much smaller percentage is anticipated. However, if a trust is seen to be generating excessive amounts of cash, the Department of Health may require that a higher rate of dividend is paid on the public dividend capital. The converse is also true, in that, if a trust has an unexpectedly large deficit in one particular year, the options of waiving or reducing the dividend for that year may be exercised, or payment of part or all of it may be postponed until a later period.

Other subsidiary controls exist to regulate the investment policy of the trust. The aim of these controls is to avoid the situation where public funds are borrowed centrally to be passed through the purchaser, as part of their cash limit, to providers where they are placed in interest bearing bank accounts. This results in a net loss to the exchequer because inevitably it costs them more to borrow than the interest that will be earned by the trust. There is no doubt that such regulatory mechanisms will be tightened as the financial discipline within NHS trusts is further developed.

Conclusion

Despite the perception in some quarters that the achievement of trust status leads automatically to much greater freedoms and an ability to undertake 'risks' and to be 'entrepreneurial', trusts are still strictly governed and regulated. The trust board has a major responsibility to determine and agree policies for the achievement of patient contracts in line with purchasers' requirements through the provision of an efficient and effective service.

Even though the introduction of trusts may be considered to allow a far more business-like approach to the delivery of health care, with terms like 'market-place', 'competitors' and 'clients' being introduced into the everyday vocabulary of the NHS, this cannot be taken to mean that any form of regulation within or without trusts is inappropriate or unwarranted. The health care market-place cannot be likened to a totally free economy and, as a result, some form of external regulation is inevitable. In fact, a range of regulatory mechanisms are in place and will continue to develop, and possibly expand, to respond to changing needs and circumstances.

Questions

1. Whilst trusts are considered to enjoy greater freedoms than directly managed units, why is regulation still necessary?
2. Appointment of the fifth executive director of a trust board is optional. Is a fifth executive director required? Assuming that the chief executive is not also fulfilling the requirement for a nursing director or medical director and that only one place is available, from which discipline should the fifth director be drawn, and why?
3. Describe and explain the main financial responsibilities of a trust, and how this differs from those of a directly managed unit. Why is there a difference?
4. A trust is only returning 4% rate of return on its assets. What options are open to it to correct this position? What are the potential knock-on effects of such actions in the short and longer term?
5. Accounting ratios are one means of providing internal and external accountability. What ratios are of value in their application to the trust financial regime? What are their relative advantages and disadvantages?

15

The potential consequences of structural change

AIMS

No organization is static and, even without the deliberate introduction of fundamental structural change, it has to develop and evolve if it is to function optimally in the changing economic environment. This at least involves adopting technological improvements as they arise, which, in the context of financial management, can be seen in the advances in information technology. The changes to the NHS which have resulted from the split between purchasers and providers have provided the impetus to introduce new management systems and technology. To a large extent methods already developed in the private sector of the economy have been used, after adapting them to the specific needs of the NHS. At present, the modifications required to implement all of the changes are at a relatively early stage of their development; they will have to be adapted and refined as time passes and their practical operation is observed.

The aims of this chapter are to consider likely developments and their impact on financial management, in particular:

- the interaction between better information and the ability of managers to use it;
- the management function;
- cost improvement programmes and the efficiency index;
- service delivery under market forces.

Information quality and uses

The White Paper, *Working for Patients*, spells out the rationale behind the reforms which are taking place in the NHS. It contains seven key objectives, one of which is:

'... to ensure that all concerned with delivering services to the patient make the best use of the resources available to them...' This desire is spelt out more clearly in the case of medical staff in the statement that the government wishes to: '... encourage further the involvement of doctors and nurses in management'. The control of resources and the participation in management of staff delivering the services requires that appropriate information is available and that they are able to use it. This identifies two branches of development which can be expected within the NHS:

- the improvement of the management information system (MIS); and
- the acquisition of resource and financial management skills by an increasing proportion of the staff.

A satisfactory information system is an essential if decision-making is to be devolved to those actually delivering health care. The intention to locate, as far as possible, decisions at the point of service delivery requires an improvement in current information systems so that staff are able to make the best use of available resources. This will be achieved by the ongoing Resource Management Initiative, the objective of which is to provide to doctors, nurses and other professional staff a detailed breakdown of the resources used in treating individual, and groups of, patients. As part of this awareness and involvement, the impact of activity on both income and costs and the consequences for budgets and actual results must be appreciated.

All decisions rely on decision-makers correctly interpreting the information they are supplied with. Data, in its crude form, can be gathered, but it is of little use until it is collated into usable information. Financial data is transformed into usable information by the accountant or finance staff, at which stage it is often merged with volume or activity measures to reflect workload or resource consumption. The accuracy of the resulting figures relies on both the financial and volume data being correct. Therefore, the managers and other professional staff responsible for the prime recording and supply of activity or volume statistics must make every effort to ensure that it is accurate. The resulting processed information, in the form of reports which combine financial and activity measures, is then passed to decision-takers

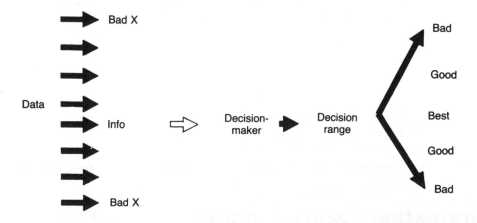

Figure 15.1 Information and the decision-maker.

who interpret it and make decisions from the range of alternatives available to them. Good information serves to limit this range to feasible alternatives and hence the likelihood of making a bad decision is reduced. The situation is presented diagramatically in Figure 15.1.

This decision-making model assumes that there are only a limited number of decisions that can be classed as 'good', but that there are an infinite number of 'bad' decisions that can be taken. The finance staff can reduce the decision range to a subset which limits the number of 'bad decision' choices, but not totally restrict them. Therefore the manager's financial awareness represents the last chance to make the correct decision. Even a good manager if presented with only 'bad' choices can only make bad decisions, and so the MIS must generate some 'good' alternatives. It can be anticipated that changes made to the MIS will have, as one objective, the production and dissemination of relevant information which will encompass the acceptable decision results and identify and exclude the bad ones.

Moving on to the uses to which information is put, the interaction between the quality of the information provided and the ability of the recipient to make optimum use of it is illustrated in Figure 15.2. There are four permutations shown in Figure 15.2, for which the four extreme points VWXY have been indicated:

- **Points W, V and Y** include at least one poor aspect as regards the quality of information and the ability of managers to use it. They are therefore obviously undesirable locations at which to operate, especially point V which demonstrates the worst of both worlds.
- **Point X** combines good financial awareness, which can be taken as a general ability to understand financial reports, including those aspects which include activity data, with a system which provides appropriate and timely information. This can be looked on as the ideal, and all organizations should have positive policies which aim to achieve it.

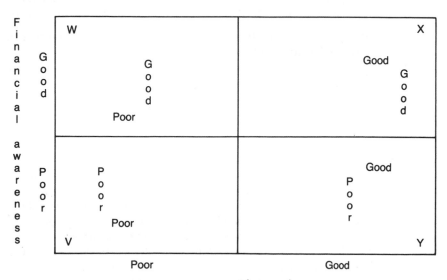

Figure 15.2 Financial awareness and MIS.

The four points V, W, X and Y tend towards the corner extremities of the grid in Figure 15.2, and it is likely that the bulk of NHS facilities lie somewhere in the middle. It is a useful exercise to attempt to determine where a particular unit or trust is positioned, possibly using an external independent assessment to pinpoint the location. Once managers know where they are on the grid, they can develop and implement plans to improve on the current position, with an initial concentration on the weaker axis. The objective is to move upwards and to the right; for example, a move from location V to W or Y represents an improvement, but a better move would be from V to X as this represents balanced development.

Experience in the year 1992–93 suggested that the balance between activity and income on an annual basis, under cash limits, has not been fully appreciated. A number of hospitals were reported to have run out of money before the end of the year while, at the same time, producing figures to show significant increases in their activity rates; in some cases reports were issued to the effect that a whole year's work had been completed in nine months of intense activity. This approach to work scheduling ignored the fact that most contracts cover a year, and so, when they have been fulfilled in terms of volume, the purchaser will not have significant remaining funds to purchase additional treatments. The rapid provision of treatment meets the desire to reduce waiting lists, but these will build up again during the period between the cash running out and the start of the new financial year when a new tranche of cash becomes available. This type of example indicates the need for a greater appreciation of the financial consequences of activity on cash flows, and the acquisition of the necessary skills can be foreseen as a likely development.

No matter where a facility is on the grid in Figure 15.2 it is able to move to a better position:

- **Financial awareness** can be enhanced through the recruitment of staff with the necessary skills, or the training of existing staff.
- **The MIS** can be improved in many ways, such as internal audits, quality circles, training, recruitment, the use of systems analysts and management consultants and better computer facilities, both in terms of hardware and software.

Even if an organization is considered to be at the optimum point X, an active policy is needed to maintain this position. Without such a policy, financially aware managers may be lost to competitors or the MIS become out of date due to lack of investment.

The conclusion to which this analysis points is that there is no room for complacency in any health unit, either DMU or trust. The environment in which the NHS now operates has the effect of indicating which units are able to manage effectively and which are not, and in those which are financially successful, it is likely that sound MIS is matched with financially aware managers at all levels.

A final matter to be aware of in the context of management information, especially when it is being used for monitoring, is the possibility of 'creative accounting'. This is best known in the case of financial reports, and has been largely countered in the NHS by the imposition of standardized accounting policies, procedures and reports. However, it can also arise in reports containing statistics, such as those dealing with activity episodes. For example, 'completed consultant episodes' (CCEs) – also known as finished consultant episodes (FCEs) – are used to measure activity, with the count increasing by one each time a consultant finishes a case. The possibility of inflating reported CCEs arises from how they are defined, and many may be logged for a single patient on the basis of a consultant merely giving advice, the transfer to a ward of a patient admitted as an emergency, and transfer between hospitals or even wards, possibly just for an investigation. In a similar way, multiple CCEs could be created by a single course of treatment such as chemotherapy which involves a number of separate attendances at a hospital, or by premature discharge followed by re-admission.

Creative accounting can be countered by drawing up definitions in increasingly restrictive ways, but the history in the accounting world is that as quickly as one area has been dealt with another arises. The tendency is for the problem to be approached in a piecemeal manner, making changes to deal with specific identified instances, and the tighter and more 'legalistically' definitions have been drawn, the more scope there has been to find ways round them. It can be anticipated that this tendency will be found in the NHS, as it has elsewhere, and so managers must be aware of its existence and not always take information at its face value.

The management function

Information is not a free good, and the general improvements in the MIS which were taking place even before the introduction of the purchaser/provider split, would, on their own, have resulted in an increase in the proportion of 'administration' employees compared with those directly delivering care to patients. This shift in the balance has been reinforced by the changes made with the introduction of the purchaser/provider split, as the relationship between these has to be administered. For example, the negotiation and supervision of contracts place extra administrative burdens on both parties.

The trend towards a higher proportion of available finance being spent on administration can be illustrated by changes in manpower. Between 1989 and 1991, the period covering the introduction of the market driven system, the fourteen RHAs in England increased the number, measured in whole time equivalents, of managers and administrative and clerical staff, while, in the same period, the number of nursing and midwifery personnel fell. The numbers involved are summarized in Table 15.1.

As is usual with any statistics, the changes shown in Table 15.1 have to be treated carefully. An initial view is that they support the contention that the NHS is being strangled in red tape and bureaucracy. However, closer analysis shows that much of the change results from the reclassification of senior staff, such as nurses, scientists

Table 15.1 Staff changes in English RHAs 1989–91

	Managers	Admin. & clerical	Nursing & midwifery
WTEs employed 30 September 1989	4 540	105 920	393 260
Change 1989–90	7 610	10 500	(8 450)
WTEs employed 30 September 1991	12 150	116 420	384 810
Percentage change	+168%	+10%	−2%

Source: Answer to Parliamentary Question.

and doctors, to administration because they have been moved to performance-related pay scales, even though doing essentially the same jobs as previously. A further distorting factor is the creation of the new group of staff called 'health care assistants'; these deal directly with patients, often supporting nurses, but are classed as administrative and clerical staff in national pay returns.

Future trends in employment patterns are likely to suggest increases in the number of managerial staff, especially at the time of creating NHS trusts, since many clinicians will participate in their management. Such a trend is fully compatible with the idea that those who can control resource usage – and hence finance – should be involved in management. A question which follows from this relates to the extent to which these individuals should then be held accountable for the results of their decisions and the activities under their control.

Therefore, the conclusions to be drawn from this brief review of trends implied from employment categories are:

- treat statistics with care – they cannot always be taken at face value;
- the increasing involvement of clinicians in management means that there is an increasing need for them to appreciate the operation of financial management.

Cost improvement programmes

Since the mid-1980s, as a result of one of the recommendations of the 1982 Griffiths Inquiry, there has been a requirement upon DHAs each year to generate part of their increased annual funding requirement internally through the adoption of formal cost improvement programmes (CIPs). This requirement is expressed as a target percentage of revenue allocation to be saved across the authority through increased efficiency and, although there may be local variations, in recent years it normally has been in the range of 1.1% to 1.3%, the higher figure often being considered to include the addition of a further target of the implementation of secondary income schemes equivalent to 0.2% of revenue allocation.

CIPs have the following features:

- The savings must be recurring and generated from specifically identified schemes. This type of saving is therefore often referred to as 'scheme specific'.
- The actual level of achievement against proposals must be capable of being monitored, must be monitored and must stand up to any form of audit.
- Schemes generally are expected actually to be 'cash releasing', i.e. the same level of work for less funding, rather than 'productivity increasing', i.e. more work for the same level of funding, otherwise funding is not actually saved and released into the system.
- Savings have to be 'genuine' and so, for example, it is not acceptable to undertake a new development with the sole intention of then stopping it as part of the CIP, nor to declare as a CIP the loss of staff posts that it was never intended to fill or fund in the first place.
- The CIP must not detrimentally affect patient volumes or standards of care.

Those involved with financial management at all levels within the NHS have a responsibility to assist in the consideration and development of each year's CIP proposals and the subsequent implementation of approved schemes. This requires a sound knowledge of how and why resources are consumed and the ability to identify and explore feasible alternative approaches to undertaking the same activity more efficiently.

The CIP initiative was introduced in the mid-1980s, well before the introduction of contracting. It was originally intended as a means of financing developments in priority areas, but the reality of the situation in recent years has been that CIP savings have been required simply to maintain purchasers' real funding levels by offsetting deficits in centrally determined annual inflation allocation increases. There is little doubt therefore that the need for CIP savings to be found will remain for many years to come. However, the concept now, and in future, has to fit into the contracting environment and the question of whether there is any need to change the process by which the required savings are identified, achieved and reported has to be addressed.

Before the introduction of the division between purchasers and providers, the likely scenario was that, at the start of a financial year, a DHA reduced in real terms the revenue allocation of each of its units and district-controlled services by an agreed percentage, such that overall the target CIP would be achieved across the authority. Each unit then had to implement schemes in the year to achieve that required level of saving. Any shortfall had to be found in the following year in addition to that next year's CIP. Such schemes tended to be agreed on a functional basis and, once identified, resulted in the budget of each functional department affected being reduced by the appropriate amount.

After the introduction of contracting, the traditional approach to CIPs has, to date, been retained. However, providers no longer receive an annual allocation of funds, but have to generate it in the form of income. As a result, the base from which reductions resulting from CIPs are measured has changed from the previous year's allocation of funds to the previous year's total income. This approach does not equate with the primary financial interest of the purchaser which is no longer concerned with the detail or analysis of functional cost within a provider, but instead with the contract price. Functional costs may well be of secondary concern in that inevitably they impact on contract price, and specific details of CIP schemes are of interest to purchasers in terms of monitoring of quality standards. However, retention of the traditional CIP approach is impeded because the purchasers have no means of assessing the impact of each CIP scheme on any individual contract price and DHAs lose direct managerial control when DMUs become NHS trusts.

An approach more suited to the changed environment in which purchasers and providers operate would be for the effect of cash-releasing schemes to be notified to purchasers in terms of their consequent **price improvements**. In other words, cost improvement programmes should be replaced with price improvement programmes, with specific price reductions replacing the identification of cost reduction schemes. A direct primary focus on price would do more to force providers to examine their costs in the competitive environment than a continual emphasis on starting the examination at the functional costs end. The final result would be the same, but represents a more logical approach to financial management in the contracting environment.

It would also assist in attempting to overcome a particular anomaly that now exists concerning CIPs. All purchasers expect an agreed level of CIP saving, and seek assurances that the total income requested from them by providers has allowed for this. However, even though the correct level of saving has been made overall, it may result in different levels of savings between purchasers, depending upon the mix of

In the financial year 19X1/X2 a provider received the following contract income:

19X1/X2	Purchaser A		Purchaser B		Total	
	Activity	Price £000	Activity	Price £000	Activity	Price £000
General surgery	3400	340	0	0	3400	340
General medicine	2000	400	1300	260	3300	660
Total	5400	740	1300	260	6700	1000

Both purchasers require a 1% CIP in 19X2/X3. Therefore, ignoring inflation, the expected contract prices each purchaser will expect to pay are:

	£000
Purchaser A (740 × 0.99)	733
Purchaser B (260 × 0.99)	257
	990

The total saving required is £10 000, and both purchasers might expect a 1% fall in their contract prices. However, to achieve the required savings, the provider implements a scheme that reduces the staffing levels on the wards that care for general surgery patients. The result is that the total cost of general surgery, and hence the total chargeable for that specialty, falls by that amount. The result of applying the revised costs to the 19X1/X2 activity levels is:

Prices revised as a result of CIPs:

19X1/X2	Purchaser A		Purchaser B		Total	
	Activity	Price £000	Activity	Price £000	Activity	Price £000
General surgery	3400	330	0	0	3400	330
General medicine	2000	400	1300	260	3300	660
Total	5400	730	1300	260	6700	990

Figure 15.3 Contract activity and costs 19X1/X2.

activity purchased and the relative impact of the savings on different contract prices. This can be illustrated by the simple example shown in Figure 15.3.

The net effect on the amount each purchaser might expect to pay in 19X2/X3 compared with what is actually charged, as computed in Figure 15.3, is:

	Procurer A £000	Procurer B £000	Total £000
Expected price after 1% saving	733	257	990
Actual price	730	260	990
Actual compared with expected: lower (higher)	3	(3)	0

Purchaser B spends the same amount in 19X2/X3 as it did in 19X1/X2, and so ends up saving nothing because it does not purchase any activity in the specialty where the saving has been made. By contrast, Purchaser A gains the full effect of the saving and is requested to pay £3000 less than it might have expected. This can be very difficult to convince purchasers of in practice and the situation would be greatly clarified if savings were identified in price terms rather than costs terms, because then purchasers would be able immediately to identify the extent of any apparent shortfall (or windfall) arising from their purchasing patterns.

The efficiency index

NHS trusts have to report regularly an efficiency index, the calculation of which is shown in Figure 15.4.

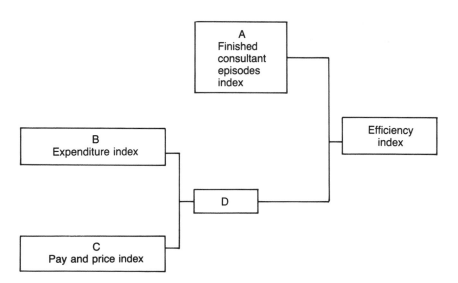

Figure 15.4 Calculation of the efficiency index.

The index works by evaluating the change in the level of activity and relating this to the impact of this change on costs. The stages in its calculation are:

- The expenditure index (B) is divided by the pay and price index (C) to reflect expenditure in real terms. A figure greater than 1 shows that the trust's costs have risen at a faster rate than would have been expected as the direct result of general costs, that is NHS-specific inflation.
- The resulting figure (D) is divided into the finished consultant episodes index (A), which is a proxy for changes in the level of activity. A figure greater than 1 shows that the level of activity has risen at a faster rate than cost increases.

The operation of the efficiency index is shown in Figure 15.5.

By combining the effects of changes in the levels of activity and costs, the efficiency index gives an overall measure which is indifferent to the functions in which the increases have actually arisen. It may be the case that some areas have become less efficient, while others have masked this at the aggregate level by making significant improvements. With further advances in the detail with which the management information system can report results, it should be possible to generate

	19X1	19X2	Index*
FCEs	16 400	16 600	1.012 (A)
Expenditure (£M)	24.000	25.500	1.063 (B)
Pay and price index	1.060 (C) (that is, a rise of 6%)		

* Calculated as 19X2/19X1.

The first step in calculating the efficiency index is to relate the increase in expenditure to that which would happen if expenditure rose in line with the general index:

$$\frac{1.063 \ (B)}{1.060 \ (C)} = 1.003 \ (D)$$

This shows that expenditure rose faster than health costs in general, that is it rose in real terms. The final index relates the increase in real expenditure to the level of activity:

$$\frac{1.012 \ (A)}{1.003 \ (D)} = 1.009$$

This is the efficiency index, and it shows that the increase in real expenditure was more than matched by the increase in the volume of activity. Another way of looking at it is that an increase in real expenditure of 0.3% was matched by an increase in activity of 1.2%.

Figure 15.5 The operation of the efficiency index.

efficiency indexes for separate parts of the organization, and so identify where efficiency is being achieved and, perhaps more importantly, where it is not.

There is a clear link between the efficiency index and CIPs, because an efficiency index greater than 1 means that more services are being delivered for the same cost, in real terms, or the same level of service at a reduced cost. The use of the efficiency index, together with its monitoring, would therefore help to facilitate a switch from CIPs to the price improvement programmes suggested above.

Market forces

The manner in which the NHS now operates has been described as a market, but it is one which has to operate in a managed way. Its main difference from what is normally understood to be a market is that it is cash limited; extra demand creates waiting lists rather than calling extra resources into the market. Left unregulated, markets can encourage suppliers to band together to create monopolies which result in higher prices, and the fact that most health services have to be supplied locally could encourage this tendency. Therefore, regulation has to be exercised to prevent NHS trusts amalgamating, so that, for example, all the DMUs in a DHA are not permitted to form a single trust.

Another feature of markets is that weak suppliers fail. Whether this is allowed to happen in the NHS is a matter of political will. By 1992 the operation of the fledgling market has already focused attention on hospitals in London, some of which, if it is left to market forces, cannot continue to operate. In the private sector, the demise of an entity is marked by the appointment of a liquidator, but such an action would not be politically acceptable. The Tomlinson Committee was established to review the health service in London, and has recommended the closure of certain facilities; this might be seen as market forces being operated, but in a structured and organized manner. The London hospitals are unlikely to be the final case where market forces point to the need for closure or major restructuring, but the final decisions on matters such as this will be subject to a political dimension.

At a more detailed level, developments can be foreseen in the type of contract used to express the market relationship. Advances in the MIS should enable a move away from block contracts towards those which link the volume of activity with the amount paid. At the extreme this is the cost per case contract, but it is unlikely that the entire service could be run on this basis, not least because of the vast flow of paperwork it would generate.

Markets operate by using information as the basis for decisions. The decision to use one facility rather than another identifies those which are offering the perceived better services, and also removes resources from those facilities which are not in favour. League tables of hospitals, introduced in the year to 31 March 1994, are intended to put information in the hands of consumers or their agents – the purchasers of health care – to help them make informed decisions. These tables initially cover such features as waiting times and cancelled operations, but there is an intention to extend them to include such aspects as cross-infection and re-admission rates.

The impact of GP fundholders

The envisaged spread of GP fundholders will increase the need for more contracts to be related to smaller groups of patients. This is because the providers will be faced by an increased number of purchasers, each dealing with a smaller number of patients on whose behalf they purchase treatment. This may be offset, to some extent, by smaller practices joining together to negotiate contracts as consortia and share administrative costs.

Another consequence of more GPs holding their own funds is the reduction of the power of DHAs, as expressed by the volume of contracts and hence funding which they are responsible for allocating. Such a trend increases the need for some form of central overview and direction of the health requirements of individual localities as the contracts placed piecemeal by a number of GPs may not, in aggregate, reflect accurately the overall health needs of an authority.

The aggregate impact of GPs holding their own funds will largely depend on the number of them which choose to follow this course. Early indications suggest that if large numbers do decide to hold their own funds, the amount of money used to purchase care from existing providers will decline. This stems from the fact that the total sum of money to be spent within the NHS is fixed, and so, when some of the money is spent in a new way, this generally means there is less available for existing activities. It has been found that GP fundholders divert funds away from existing providers in three ways:

- **Surpluses are retained** in the practice and used to fund developments, possibly in the form of enhancing fixed assets.
- **Administration costs** of GP fundholders take a higher proportion of the funds available to procure treatment than is the case with DHAs, the former accounting for about 5% while the latter takes only around 3%.
- **Direct provision of services** occurs where GPs channel the provision of health care to their patients through novel routes; in some cases this is the GP's own limited company, although the future of such arrangements is under review.

The list of treatments which the GP can provide directly is limited and tends to cover relatively inexpensive cases; the overall impact is also limited because of the relatively small proportion of fundholding GPs. However, any restriction on the volume of funds fed into the existing pattern of provision means that both DMUs and trusts are faced with the possibility of reduced potential income. The impact of lower income on organizations with a high level of fixed costs is to at least increase the average cost per unit of throughput. This leads to a reduction in competitive advantage as a result of higher prices which may cause purchasers to purchase treatment elsewhere. In this way, a spiral of decline may be initiated. Even if this position is not reached, DMUs and trusts are likely to have to learn how to function and adapt without the availability of the marginal, uncommitted funds which have been eroded by the emergence of GP fundholders.

One benefit which GP fundholders may bring is to enforce cash management on providers. In the early stages of the scheme's operation it was found that GPs spread their expenditure over the whole year, and so tended to have funds still available after the main purchasers had spent all of theirs. These funds are eagerly sought by providers to finance the gap between the early completion of their DHA contracts and the new financial year.

The emergence of explicit decisions

The ability to spend money, especially on health care, is virtually unlimited, but is constrained by the amount of money available. In the case of the NHS, the volume of funds to be spent each year is set by the government and imposes the need to decide exactly what set of services are to be provided. In the same way as any organization, or individual, operating under financial limits has to make choices, the decision to spend a given sum of money in a particular way precludes all the other possible ways it could have been spent.

In the private sector, the operation of market forces allocates the available funds, and it is assumed that national utility is maximized as each individual acquires that set of goods and services which maximizes his or her own well-being. In this way, the total amount of money spent on, say, televisions is determined by the market. If a consumer decides that a television is more desirable than a new carpet, then the demand for televisions increases and the amount spent on them grows; conversely, the demand for carpets falls, and the amount spent on them declines.

The supply of health care to the general population is not left to market forces as political forces have dictated that it would not result in an equitable distribution. This is because a proportion of the population would not have, at a given time, the resources to be able to buy the care needed. Therefore, the NHS is, for the most part, funded from general taxation and care provided free at the point of delivery.

In the absence of market forces, extra demand for NHS services does not result in a reallocation of resources from other possible items of expenditure to health care; instead, if it cannot be met from improved efficiency or growth money, it leads to longer waiting lists. The patient is free to make a market choice and purchase health care in the private sector, which reduces the demands placed on the NHS. However, even though considerable use is made of private medical services, it has not had the effect of cutting down the demand for NHS services to the extent that it can be met in full.

The fact that the amount of health care provided by the NHS is not determined by market forces means that some other mechanism has to be developed to convert the funding provided into specific treatments. An alternative way of looking at this is that, whatever mechanism is used, the decisions made will result in the treatment of a number of patients being postponed, perhaps indefinitely. Ideally, the NHS would use its funds in such a way as to maximize an index reflecting the general health of the population, but such an index does not exist in a form which could make it part of the decision model. Instead, purchasers use the funds they are given to purchase the care which is considered most appropriate to the population they serve. The fact that there are a number of providers means that competition to meet the requirements of the purchasers drives down costs.

Controlling the relationship between the purchasers and providers by means of priced contracts has the effect that the decisions facing purchasers are made explicit and the opportunity cost of each choice can be seen. The selection of a particular set of treatments can be weighed against an alternative set with the same cost. However, the decision as to which represents the 'better' set of treatments relies on deciding which one gives the greater health gain, and, especially as it approaches the use of marginal funds, informed subjective judgement has to be used. Therefore, the adoption of increasingly sophisticated financial management techniques to aid the contracting process has enabled greater accuracy to be introduced to the cost side of the cost–benefit equation, but the benefit side still lacks the degree of precision needed if it is to determine the selection of the services to be purchased.

Activity and its financial consequences

When activity is undertaken, resources are consumed, and resources cost money. The resource may be intangible, for example an employee's time, or tangible, like drugs and dressings. The introduction of capital charges has had the effect that capital assets, which were once free goods, now have a cost associated with them. The process of financial management links resource consumption with its financial consequences and also enables an organization to measure the extent to which it is operating within the constraints to which it is subject. In the NHS, at the overall level for each DMU or trust, these are as follows:

- **Cash** inflows and outflows reported in the cash flow statement have to balance, subject to any surplus or deficit agreed by a trust as an external financing limit.
- **Resource** inflows and outflows, as measured in the income and expenditure account, have to remain broadly in balance.

A system of budgetary control is needed to monitor actual results against those expected on a regular basis and enable corrective action to be taken if it becomes clear that financial objectives are not being achieved. On the cost side, the overall position, in terms of both cash and expenditure, is reached as the aggregate of all the individual decisions made to consume resources. It is therefore important that those responsible for the level of consumption have sufficient financial awareness to be able to understand the impact of their decisions on the overall results.

Purchasers are free to decide from which facilities they will buy health care; they can use local DMUs and trusts, ones which are further afield, and the private sector. The decision of which ones to employ is based on a number of factors, but the main factor is expected to be value for money. At a more detailed level, the cost of different procedures, the length of the waiting list, and acceptability to patients are relevant. The consequences of this arrangement are as follows:

- Providers have to be 'competitive' and actively work to attract contracts. This will involve keeping prices as low as possible, subject to a quality threshold, and seeking to reduce waiting times.
- The private sector offers a point of reference on pricing. Where the private sector offers to carry out work at a lower cost, then it can be given the work, and, where it provides services not currently available in the NHS, then potential savings from internal provision can be easily identified. For example, early in 1993 the NHS paid a private psychiatric hospital £5500 per week for each patient; the opinion was expressed by a consultant that the NHS could provide the service more cheaply, and so the service provided by the private sector should be switched to the NHS.
- The level of a facility's income is not guaranteed from one year to the next; one year a new contract may be gained, and the next year lost. Also, the full amount of income for a particular year only becomes apparent as the year progresses; for example, one area of uncertainty is the number of ECRs treated. It is possible that a minimum base load can be identified, but, with the high level of fixed costs

incurred in providing treatment, optimum efficiency is reached at or near full capacity. Living with an indeterminate level of income means that costs have to be managed carefully to ensure that they do not exceed income. This requires resource consumers to be aware of cost behaviour and how to flex expenditure to balance it with income.

Conclusion

At the time of writing, the reforms taking place in the NHS are still at a relatively early stage in their development. Some trends, such as improvements in MIS, can already be seen, but other, as yet unforeseen, consequences are also likely. To meet the challenges which the latter type represent, individuals who are responsible for consuming resources in the NHS, and hence spending its funds, must have a grasp of financial management. They must be aware both of the detailed level – for example, how such figures in reports as 'income' are generated – and at the overall level when considering such matters as how market forces are expressed through contracts and the consequences of negotiating different types.

The general conclusion from this analysis is that individual parts of the NHS will, in future, be living in a less certain world, although they are bounded by specific constraints, such as making a set level of return on capital employed. Financial management provides the tools to enable the operators to optimize how well they survive. An organization which has financially aware staff can be expected to survive better than one where individuals are not aware of the consequences of their actions for the organization as a whole.

The techniques and procedures explained in this book constitute an introduction to the practicalities of financial management in the new NHS, but the everyday detail will be more intricate than the examples provided. However, this book provides the foundations required by individuals to enhance their financial awareness to enable them to adapt to future developments as they arise.

Appendix:
Suggested solutions to selected questions

Note: The following solutions are provided for those questions marked in the text with an asterisk.

Chapter 3

1. (a) Depreciation charge £154.
   Written down value £935.
   (b) If the asset were purchased by a non-NHST, capital charges would include interest as well as depreciation, and would total £197.

   The above values are calculated as follows:

Quarter	1 £000	2 £000	3 £000	4 £000	Total £000
Replacement value					
Opening value	–	1010.00	1030.00	1030.00	
Purchases	1000.00	–	–	–	
Indexation	10.00	20.00	–	70.00	
Closing value	1010.00	1030.00	1030.00	1100.00	
Depreciation					
Opening value	–	–	51.52	103.02	
Quarterly charge	–	50.50	51.50	51.50	153.50
Accumulated charge	–	50.50	103.02	154.52	
Indexation	–	1.02	–	10.50	

Closing value		51.52	103.02	165.02	
Book value	1010.00	978.48	926.98	934.98	
Interest charge	–	15.15	14.68	13.91	43.74
Total charge					197.24

Notes:
1. Interest and depreciation are not charged in the quarter of acquisition, but the asset is indexed.
2. The indexation is carried out by multiplying the value to be indexed by:

$$\frac{\text{Closing index} - \text{Opening index}}{\text{Opening index}}$$

3. Each quarter's opening replacement value and accumulated charge are indexed to arrive at closing values at current value.
4. The depreciation charge for each quarter is the opening current value divided by the asset's life in quarters.
5. The closing book value is found by subtracting the closing accumulated depreciation from the closing replacement value.

3. £9 450 000 (£800 000 + £9 600 000 − £950 000)

Chapter 5

2.

	19X5 £000	19X6 £000
Working capital	775	450
Working capital ratio	2.3 : 1	1.5 : 1
Liquidity ratio	0.8 : 1	0.4 : 1

All values show a deterioration. The fact that a fall has taken place is not always an indication of problems as the fall may have been from an excellent position to a good one. However, in this case the lack of cash and high level of creditors suggests impending problems.

Chapter 6

6. The finance director has taken all costs and assumed that they are directly related to activity, i.e. that they are variable. This is not the case. Most costs will be fixed, and even where costs are apportioned the cost centre involved is unlikely to face a significantly lower total cost bill if the bed number reduces on just one ward. In such cases it is assumed that most departments will face the cost structure 75% fixed and 25% variable.

Revised ward costs for 19X2 are as follows.

- **Medical salaries.** The consultant and registrar will still need to be employed, but the number of house officers could feasibly be reduced if a suitable on-call rota could be established. This will result in additional on-call sessions, therefore the saving would not be equivalent to one house officer. In any event medical posts are generally fixed in the short term, therefore no saving will result.

- **Nursing costs.** Senior nurses will still need to be in post and any pro-rata reduction in RGN auxiliaries is conditional upon adequate cover being provided on the ward. There may be a saving of RGNs and auxiliaries. This will be possible where bank nurses are used or if cross cover is feasible, i.e. where specialist skills are not required. Given the total number of nursing staff employed, 22 working 37-hour weeks, and the need to provide 24-hour cover, the current level only allows for just less than five staff at any one time. This is clearly as close to the limit as is feasible. Therefore no reduction in staff will be forthcoming.
- **Medical equipment.** This figure presumably relates to miscellaneous minor purchases which do not fall within the definition of capital. Equipment is acquired for all patients, not just the ten beds no longer utilized. Therefore this is unlikely to change.
- **Pharmacy.** Perhaps the drugs issued is a true variable cost as only patients are prescribed drugs. However, included in this apportionment will be the fixed costs of running the pharmacy and while the ward may achieve a saving of £11 500 it is unlikely that the costs faced by the pharmacy will fall by this amount. The 75:25 rule is applied to give an estimated saving of £2875. (In practice the 'rule' may be more of the order of 80:20 for departments employing mainly professional and technical staff.)
- **Pathology.** The same concept as pharmacy. While less requests will be processed the cost structure of the pathology laboratory will have a high fixed proportion, especially staff and capital charges. So while the ward may save £3175 the trust's overall costs will remain largely unaffected. If only 25% of the pathology laboratories costs are variable then only this proportion will be saved.
- **Radiology.** The same argument as pharmacy and pathology applies. Bear in mind that the reduction in patient numbers will mean that the total costs will be borne by a smaller apportionment base and therefore cost per X-ray request will rise to other radiology department users.
- **Catering.** The catering department is also unlikely to face a significant reduction in costs as a result of ten less meals to prepare. Provisions costs may be marginally affected, but staffing and other non-pay costs will remain unchanged.
- **Cleaning.** The floor area will not change and the whole ward will need to be adequately cleaned despite the decrease in beds.
- **Heating and lighting.** As with cleaning the whole area will still need to be heated and well lit.
- **Estate management.** Once again no change in floor area means no change in cost.
- **General management.** As administration is based on employee numbers some reduction in the apportionment can be expected. However, in reality the administration department will probably still have to perform exactly the same tasks as before and so the cost implications will be minimal.

Any saving appears to be minimal and this needs to be compared against the potential income loss in terms of the lower number of patients treated. In any event the finance director has assumed a full occupancy on the ward, which is not a realistic assumption for any acute service. A 75% level of occupancy may be quite normal in which case there may be no real saving whatsoever. An acute ward with 80% occupancy is probably operating at or near maximum efficiency given the time required for patient turnover.

7. First, variable and fixed costs for 19X3 need to be determined:

Variable costs

	£
Catering	43 800
Laundry	8 800
Dietetics	3 200
Physiotherapy	5 700
Radiography	9 200
Pathology	7 500
Pharmacy	9 400
Total variable costs (at 19X2 prices)	87 600
Inflation factor	5%
19X3 estimate	91 980

Occupancy level 50% × 24 = 12 × 365 days = 4380 patient days
Variable cost per patient day = 91 980/4380 = £21

Fixed costs

	£
Domestic	12 000
Portering	8 000
General management	15 000
Estate management	7 000
	42 000
Uplift factor	5%
	44 100
Rates	50 000
Capital charges	80 000
	174 100

Stepped costs

Patient numbers	Nurses required	Nursing budget £
0 to 4	5	100 000
5 to 8	10	200 000
9 to 12	15	300 000
13 to 16	20	400 000
17 to 20	25	500 000
21 to 24	30	600 000

Flexed budget for 19X3

Patient numbers	Fixed costs £	Stepped costs £	Variable costs £	Total costs £	Total income £	Surplus (deficit) £
4	174 100	100 000	30 660	304 760	189 800	(114 960)
8	174 100	200 000	61 320	435 420	379 600	(55 820)
12	174 100	300 000	91 980	566 080	569 400	3 320
16	174 100	400 000	122 640	696 740	759 200	62 460
20	174 100	500 000	153 300	827 400	949 000	121 600
24	174 100	600 000	183 960	958 060	1 138 800	180 740

Comment

The current level of charges will produce a small surplus for the unit if occupancy levels remain unchanged. However, the forecasts assume a level of inflation of 5% and the budgeted surplus is only half a percent more than total costs. This is clearly a highly sensitive position and management needs to consider either increasing the charges for the coming year or ensuring a higher utilization of the facility.

Chapter 7

3. **Note:** for the purposes of presentation, all example calculations are rounded to either the nearest £1000 or the nearest £100.

(a) **The single step-down method.** Costs are apportioned directly to the wards using a suitable basis. A suggested basis for each heading or group of headings is as follows.

- **Medical staff and nursing staff.** These are direct costs, allocated directly to the wards.
- **Pathology and radiology.** Apportioned on the basis of deaths and discharges in each ward group. The cost of drugs issued to the radiology department is not accounted for in this apportionment (see drugs below).
- **Drugs.** The total drug cost is apportioned pro rata to the relative drug use by each ward group, ignoring issues to any other department. The cost per ward group is therefore calculated by dividing their drug cost by £750 000 and not £800 000, e.g.

  General surgery = (350/750) × £800 000 = £373 333

- **Pharmacy staff.** Apportioned on the basis of drugs issues, i.e. using £250 000 in the previous equation, rather than £800 000.
- **Housekeeping.** Apportioned on the relative floor areas of each ward group. For example:

  General medicine = (2000/(2000 + 4000 + 1000)) × £300 000 = £86 000

- **Rates, energy and works maintenance.** Apportioned on the basis of relative volumes of each ward group. For example:

  Rates for obstetrics = (3500/(7000 + 14 000 + 3500)) × £200 000
  = £29 000

Table A7.1 Summary of costs using single step-down method

Heading	Basis	General medicine £000	General surgery £000	Obstetrics £000	Total £000
Medical staff	Direct	200	350	150	700
Nursing staff	Direct	750	950	450	2150
Pathology	D & D	150	300	150	600
Radiology	D & D	113	225	113	450
Drugs	Issues	320	373	107	800
Pharmacy staff	Issues	100	117	33	250
Housekeeping	Floor area	86	171	43	300
Rates	Volume	57	114	29	200
Energy	Volume	43	86	21	150
Works maint'ce	Volume	51	103	26	180
Grounds	D & D	13	25	13	50
Management	Employees	54	76	40	170
Total costs		1936	2890	1174	6000

- **Grounds and gardens.** Whichever basis is used is likely to be arbitrary. In this case deaths and discharges is as good a choice as any. It is probably equally as valid to have based it upon relative employee numbers, or direct costs, or even as a final mark-up based on all other costs.
- **Management.** Another less than straightforward choice. In this case relative staff numbers in each ward group have been used. For example:

General surgery = $(85/(60 + 85 + 45)) \times £170\,000 = £76\,000$

The calculations are summarized in Table A7.1. Simply dividing each of these total costs (which are expressed in £000s) by deaths and discharges for each ward group produces the cost per D & D, as follows:

Cost per death/discharge	Gen. med. £	Gen. surg. £	Obs. £	Total £
	1936	1445	1174	1500

(b) **The multiple step-down method.** The steps shown in Table A7.2 are a slight variation of those illustrated in Figure 7.12, whereby an additional 'step' to apportion both drug and pharmacy costs on the basis of actual issues is introduced. Direct costs are allocated to each department and are then apportioned down through each level in turn, using a suitable basis. A suggested basis for each heading or group of headings is as follows. (Note that costs have been rounded to the nearest £100 in the illustrative calculations below.)

- **Energy and rates.** Apportioned on the basis of relative volumes of each department group. For example:

Housekeeping energy = $(75/28\,000) \times £150\,000 = £400$

- **Grounds and gardens.** This could easily be directly costed against just the ward groups by simply using deaths and discharges as the basis. However, assume that relative staff numbers are to be used. For example:

Works maintenance = $(15/345) \times £50\,000 = £2200$

Table A7.2 Summary of costs using multiple step-down method

Heading	Basis	General medicine £000	General surgery £000	Obstetrics £000	Pathology £000	Radiology £000	Pharmacy £000	Works maintenance £000	House-keeping £000	Management £000	Total £000
Energy	Volume	37.5	75.0	18.8	6.0	8.0	2.0	0.9	0.4	1.3	150.0
Rates	Volume	50.0	100.0	25.0	8.0	10.7	2.7	1.3	0.5	1.8	200.0
Grounds	Employees	8.7	12.3	6.5	6.5	5.8	2.2	2.2	4.3	1.4	50.0
Sub-total		96.2	187.3	50.3	20.6	24.5	6.9	4.4	5.3	4.6	400.0
Direct costs								180.0	300.0	170.0	650.0
Total for apportionment*		96.2	187.3	50.3	20.6	24.5	6.9	184.4*	305.3*	174.6*	1050.0
Works maintenance	Volume	46.9	93.9	23.5	7.5	10.1	2.5	(184.4)			(0.0)
Housekeeping	Floor area	74.5	148.9	37.2	16.8	22.3	5.6		(305.3)		0.0
Management	Employees	36.1	51.2	27.1	27.1	24.1	9.0			(174.6)	(0.0)
Sub-total		253.7	481.3	138.1	72.0	81.0	24.0	0.0	0.0	0.0	1050.0
Drugs	Issues	300.0	350.0	100.0		50.0					800.0
Direct costs							250.0				250.0
Total for apportionment*		553.7	831.3	238.1	72.0	131.0	274.0*	0.0	0.0	0.0	2100.0
Pharmacy	Issues	102.7	119.9	34.2	0.0	17.1	(274.0)				0.0
Sub-total		656.4	951.1	272.3	72.0	148.1	0.0				2100.0
Direct costs					600.0	450.0					1050.0
Total for apportionment*		656.4	951.1	272.3	672.0*	598.1*	0.0				3150.0
Pathology	D & D	168.0	336.0	168.0	(672.0)						0.0
Radiology	D & D	149.5	299.1	149.5		(598.1)					0.0
Pharmacy	Issues	974.0	1586.2	589.8	0.0	0.0	0.0				3150.0
Direct costs (Med & Nursing)		950.0	1300.0	600.0	0.0	0.0	0.0				2850.0
Total costs for		1924.0	2886.2	1189.8	0.0	0.0	0.0	0.0	0.0	0.0	6000.0
Cost per death/discharge		£1924	£1443	£1190							

Note that the divider is 345 and not 350 employees because the staff employed in the grounds and gardens department have to be excluded from the calculation to avoid a loop situation.

The calculation can now move to the next 'step'.

- **Works maintenance.** By applying the steps shown in Figure 7.12 this is apportioned across the three diagnostic departments (pathology, radiology and pharmacy) and the three ward groups on the basis of their relative volumes. For example:

$$\text{Radiology} = (1500/(7000 + 14\,000 + 3500 + 1125 \\ + 1500 + 375)) \times £184\,400 = £10\,100$$

Remember that the total amount apportioned is the sum of the direct costs plus costs apportioned to the department in previous steps – in this case the works department costs include £4400, being costs apportioned on the previous step.

- **Housekeeping.** As with the previous heading, but apportioned on the basis of relative floor areas. For example:

$$\text{Pathology} = (450/(2000 + 4000 + 1000 + 450 + 600 + 150)) \\ \times £305\,300 = £16\,800$$

- **Management.** As with the previous heading, but apportioned on the basis of employee numbers. For example:

$$\text{Pharmacy} = (15/(60 + 85 + 45 + 45 + 40 + 15)) \times £174\,600 = £9000$$

The calculation now moves to the next step, that of apportioning the drug and pharmacy costs. This step has to be introduced because part of the drug cost has been incurred by a department that is not in the final level, i.e. radiology.

- **Drugs.** Apportioned on the basis of actual issues.

- **Pharmacy.** Apportioned on the basis of drug issues (in effect as an 'oncost'). Note that the costs previously apportioned to the department have to be included in the total cost for apportionment. For example:

$$\text{Obstetrics} = 100/800 \times £274\,000 = £34\,200$$

The calculation now proceeds to the next step.

- **Pathology.** Apportioned on the basis of deaths and discharges. For example:

$$\text{General medicine} = (1000/(1000 + 2000 + 1000)) \times £672\,000 \\ = £168\,000$$

A much better basis would have been weighted units of work by ward group, if available.

- **Radiology.** As per pathology. For example:

$$\text{General surgery} = (2000/(1000 + 2000 + 1000)) \times £598\,100 = £299\,100$$

Chapter 8

5.

	£		Responsible manager
Staff variances:			
Rate	2400 × (1.75 − 1.50) = 600	A	Pathologist
Efficiency	1.50 × (2500 − 2400) = 150	F	Clinician
	450	A	
Non-staff variances:			
Price	2400 × (0.80 − 1.00) = 480	F	Supplies
Usage	1.00 × (2500 − 2400) = 100	F	Clinician
	580	F	

Comment

The pathology manager is not to be congratulated as the overall favourable variance of £130 is made up of favourable variances of (150 + 480 + 100) £730 attributable to clinicians and the supplies department while the pathology department has performed badly with a £600 adverse variance nearly cancelling the efficiencies gained elsewhere.

Chapter 9

5. (a) The standard cost equals the total planned cost of the department divided by the associated planned workload level, i.e.:

	Cost £000	Units 000	Standard cost £
Staff	300	300	1.00
Consumables	100	300	0.33
O'heads/recharges	200	300	0.67
Total	600	300	2.00

The budgets for 19X6/X7 should look similar to the following. A single line for overheads/recharges inward is show for simplicity:

Pathology department budget 19X6/X7

	Units	Budget £000
Direct costs:		
Staff costs		300
Consumables		100
O'heads/recharges		200
	300 000	600

Recharges outward:

General surgery	(80 000)	(160)
Thoracic surgery	(50 000)	(100)
General medicine	(60 000)	(120)
Acute care of elderly	(30 000)	(60)
Child health	(45 000)	(90)
Gynaecology	(35 000)	(70)
	(300 000)	(600)
Total budget		0

Thoracic surgery budget 19X6/X7

	Units	Budget £000
Direct costs		700
Overheads etc.		150
Path. tests from outside labs		50
Pathology recharges	50 000	100
		1000

(b) The financial impact of the switch to the external laboratory can be calculated as follows:

(i) **Thoracic surgery directorate.** The additional cost incurred for external tests is the number of tests multiplied by the cost per test:

$$1500 \times £30.00 = £45\,000$$

(ii) **Pathology department.** The saving is not £15 000, because only the variable costs will be saved in the short term. Staff and overhead/recharges inward costs are fixed in the short term. Thus the only savings in the short term will stem from a reduced level of use of consumables.

Units saved = 1500 × 20 = 30 000		(30 000)
Standard cost per unit (consumables)	£	0.33
Saving =	£	(10 000)

The result of this action is that the trust is actually £35 000 worse off (£10 000 − £45 000), and not £15 000 better off. If the CD were then to spend the £15 000, the trust would be £50 000 worse off overall. This represents the pathology department fixed costs no longer recovered through the internal charging mechanism, namely 1500 tests multiplied by the fixed costs element of the standard cost, i.e. £1.00 + £0.67:

$$30\,000 \text{ units} \times £1.67 = £50\,000$$

Chapter 11

5. (a) Table A11.1 shows the revised cost schedule which results from taking 19X4/X5 costs as the basis for costing the 19X5/X6 contracts, and uplifting them for the inflation shown in Table 11.8, line A.

Each entry is calculated by uplifting the figures in each column of Table 11.7 by the relevant inflation percentage.

Initial contract prices, shown in Table A11.2, can then be calculated by dividing total planned cost by planned activity, as set out in Table 11.8, line C.

Table A11.3 shows the effect of applying the initial contract prices to each purchaser's anticipated activity levels, as set out in Table 11.8, line C.

(b) The impact of each change can be determined in turn, by starting with the position set out in Table 11.7.

Step 1

Adjust for the CIP by reducing the costs recharged from pathology to general surgery. The amount shown for general surgery recharges under the heading Fixed costs, Staff, reduces from £200 000 to £125 000.

Step 2

Adjust for the amended activity levels by increasing or reducing the variable costs in proportion to the change. Only the total activity in each specialty is relevant to this calculation, namely:

	General surgery	General medicine	Total
Initial assumption	6000.0	8000.0	14 000.0
Final agreement	6900.0	7600.0	14 500.0

For example, the calculation for General medicine, Radiology, Variable non-staff costs is:

Table 11.7 amount	£	300 000.0
Divide by initial activity assumption	÷	8 000.0
Cost per patient	=	37.5
Multiply by final activity	×	7 600.0
Adjusted costs	£	285 000.0

Uplift to reflect the agreed rates of inflation for inclusion within the calculations. For example, continuing the above example:

Adjusted costs, pre-inflation	£285 000.0
Inflation @ 4.00%	£ 11 400.0
Total	£296 400.0

The combined impact of these changes are summarized in Tables A11.4, A11.5 and A11.6. A number of points may be noted, primarily:

- An increased demand of 1000 general surgery patients by Purchaser A has resulted in income increasing by approximately £400 000.
- A reduced demand of 500 general medicine patients by Purchaser B has resulted in income reducing by approximately £300 000.
- Purchaser C's activity levels have remained unchanged, but income has fallen by approximately £100 000.

The specific impact of each of the changes on these movements can only be determined by calculating each effect separately.

Table A11.1 Planned costs 19X5/X6

Dept/Directorate	Fixed costs		Variable costs		Total costs £000
	Staff £000	Non-staff £000	Staff £000	Non-staff £000	
General surgery:					
Direct costs	615.0	104.5	102.5	103.5	925.5
Overheads/recharges:					
Pathology	205.0	104.5	0.0	103.5	413.0
Radiology	153.8	156.8	0.0	207.0	517.5
Pharmacy	153.8	52.3	0.0	310.5	516.5
Works/utilities	51.3	104.5	0.0	51.8	207.5
Housekeeping	51.3	20.9	0.0	0.0	72.2
Catering	71.8	156.8	0.0	51.8	280.3
Management	133.3	31.4	0.0	0.0	164.6
	1435.0	731.5	102.5	828.0	3097.0
General medicine:					
Direct costs	1025.0	156.8	51.3	310.5	1543.5
Overheads/recharges:					
Pathology	358.8	209.0	0.0	155.3	723.0
Radiology	205.0	209.0	0.0	310.5	724.5
Pharmacy	205.0	104.5	0.0	414.0	723.5
Works/utilities	71.8	135.9	0.0	103.5	311.1
Housekeeping	51.3	20.9	0.0	0.0	72.2
Catering	102.5	188.1	0.0	72.5	363.1
Management	153.8	31.4	0.0	0.0	185.1
	2173.0	1055.5	51.3	1366.2	4645.9
Total all costs	3608.0	1787.0	153.8	2194.2	7742.9

Table A11.2 Initial contract prices 19X5/X6

	General surgery	General medicine	Total
Total cost (£000) (Table A11.1)	3097	4646	7743
Activity (Table 11.8)	6000	8000	14000
Contract price (£)	516	581	

Table A11.3 Income analysis by purchaser (Table 11.8 activity multiplied by Table A11.2 contract price)

	General surgery £000	General medicine £000	Total £000
Purchaser A	1548.5	3077.9	4626.4
Purchaser B	516.2	1451.8	1968.0
Purchaser C	929.1	116.1	1045.2
Purchaser D	103.2	0.0	103.2
	3097.0	4645.9	7742.9

Table A11.4 Revised planned costs 19X5/X6

Dept/Directorate	Fixed costs		Variable costs		Total costs £000
	Staff £000	Non-staff £000	Staff £000	Non-staff £000	
General surgery:					
Direct costs	612.0	108.0	117.3	119.6	956.9
Overheads/recharges:					
Pathology	127.5	108.0	0.0	119.6	355.1
Radiology	153.0	162.0	0.0	239.2	554.2
Pharmacy	153.0	54.0	0.0	358.8	565.8
Works/utilities	51.0	108.0	0.0	59.8	218.8
Housekeeping	51.0	21.6	0.0	0.0	72.6
Catering	71.4	162.0	0.0	59.8	293.2
Management	132.6	32.4	0.0	0.0	165.0
	1351.5	756.0	117.3	956.8	3181.6
General medicine:					
Direct costs	1020.0	162.0	48.5	296.4	1526.9
Overheads/recharges:					
Pathology	357.0	216.0	0.0	148.2	721.2
Radiology	204.0	216.0	0.0	296.4	716.4
Pharmacy	204.0	108.0	0.0	395.2	707.2
Works/utilities	71.4	140.4	0.0	98.8	310.6
Housekeeping	51.0	21.6	0.0	0.0	72.6
Catering	102.0	194.4	0.0	69.2	365.6
Management	153.0	32.4	0.0	0.0	185.4
	2162.4	1090.8	48.5	1304.2	4605.8
Total all costs	3513.9	1846.8	165.8	2261.0	7787.4

Table A11.5 Revised contract prices 19X5/X6

	General surgery	General medicine	Total
Total cost (£000) (Table A11.4)	3182	4606	7787
Activity (Table 11.9)	6900	7600	14 500
Contract price (£)	461	606	

Table A11.6 Income analysis by purchaser (Table 11.9 activity multiplied by Table A11.5 contract price)

	General surgery £000	General medicine £000	Total £000
Purchaser A	1844.4	3211.9	5056.4
Purchaser B	461.1	1212.1	1673.2
Purchaser C	830.0	121.2	951.2
Purchaser D	46.1	60.6	106.7
	3181.6	4605.8	7787.4

Further reading

Buxton, M., Packwood, T. and Keen, J. (1989) *Resource Management: Process and Progress*, Health Economics Research Group, Brunel University.

Buxton, M., Packwood, T. and Keen, J. (1991) *Final report of the Brunel University Evaluation of Resource Management*, Brunel University.

CIPFA (1992) *Index to Health Authority Manual for Accounts*.

CIPFA (1993) *Explaining ECR Price Differences*.

CIPFA (1993) *Guide to Good Practice – Costing: Outpatients*.

Commons Health Committee (1992) *NHS Trusts: Interim Conclusions and Proposals for Future Enquiries*, HMSO.

DHSS (1986) *Health Service Management – Resource Management (Management Budgeting) in Health Authorities*, Health Notice (86)34.

DoH (1989) *Working for Patients*, HMSO. This has nine associated working papers:
1. Self Governing Hospitals
2. Funding and Contracts for Hospital Services
3. Practice Budgets for General Medical Practitioners
4. Indicative Prescribing Budgets for General Medical Practitioners
5. Capital Charges
6. Medical Audit
7. NHS Consultants: Appointments, Contracts and Distinction Awards
8. Implications for Family Practitioners Committees
9. Capital Charges: Funding Issues.

Ellwood, S. (1992) *Cost Methods for NHS Healthcare Contracts*, Chartered Institute of Management Accountants.

Harrison, A. (ed.) *Health Care UK 1991*, King's Fund Institute (this is an annual publication).

Health Economics Research Unit (1992) *DRGs: The Road to Hospital Efficiency*, Aberdeen University.

Healthcare Financial Management Association, *Guide to Good Practice – Costing: Costing for Purchasers, Supporting Health Strategy*, CIPFA.

Hunter D. (1993) *Rationing Dilemmas in Healthcare*, NAHAT.

Jenkins, L., McKee, M. and Sanderson, H. (1990) *DRGs – A Guide to Grouping and Interpretation*, CASPE Research.

King's Fund (1992) *A Foothold for Fundholding*, King's Fund Institute.

Körner, E. (1984) *Sixth Report of the Steering Group on Health Service Information*, HMSO.

National Association of Health Authorities and Trusts (1992) *Financial Survey of Health Authorities and Provider Units*, NAHAT.

National Association of Health Authorities and Trusts (1992) *Priority Setting in Purchasing: Some Practical Guidelines*, NAHAT.

Newchurch and Company (1993) *Third Newchurch Guide to NHS Trusts*, London.

NHS Management Board (1989) *Case-Mix Management System: Core Specification*.

NHSME (1990) *Capital Charges Manual*.

NHSME, *Financial Proformas* (regular publication of current requirements).

NHSME, *Manual of Accounts* (regular publication of current requirements).

NHSME, *NHS Trust Finance Manual* (regular publication of current requirements).

Perrin, J. (1988) *Resource Management in the NHS*, Chapman & Hall, London.

Prowle, M., Jones, T. and Shaw, J. (1989) *Working for Patients: The Financial Agenda*, Chartered Association of Certified Accountants, London.

Tomlinson, B. (1992) *Report of the Inquiry into London's Health Service, Medical Education and Research*, HMSO.

Index